Amira Kikly
Sabra Jaâfoura

Management of early caries lesions

Amira Kikly
Sabra Jaâfoura

Management of early caries lesions

Management of early carious lesions: Minimally invasive approach

ScienciaScripts

Imprint

Any brand names and product names mentioned in this book are subject to trademark, brand or patent protection and are trademarks or registered trademarks of their respective holders. The use of brand names, product names, common names, trade names, product descriptions etc. even without a particular marking in this work is in no way to be construed to mean that such names may be regarded as unrestricted in respect of trademark and brand protection legislation and could thus be used by anyone.

Cover image: www.ingimage.com

This book is a translation from the original published under ISBN 978-620-6-71282-4.

Publisher:
Sciencia Scripts
is a trademark of
Dodo Books Indian Ocean Ltd. and OmniScriptum S.R.L publishing group

120 High Road, East Finchley, London, N2 9ED, United Kingdom
Str. Armeneasca 28/1, office 1, Chisinau MD-2012, Republic of Moldova, Europe
Printed at: see last page
ISBN: 978-620-7-71420-9

Management of early carious lesions: Minimally invasive approach

Table of contents

Introduction

In recent decades, the management of carious lesions in dentistry has evolved from invasive dentistry to microinvasive dentistry, which strives to keep the dental organ in the mouth as long as possible, at the cost of minimal surgical intervention and maximum, constant prevention for patients.

Traditionally, caries was seen as a lesion that needed to be treated surgically, by eradicating the demineralized tooth structure and replacing it with an inert material that would restore the tooth to its original appearance. However, this type of treatment cured the signs and symptoms of carious disease and restored the form, function and aesthetics of the teeth, but in no way prevented the development of new carious lesions. Consequently, it offered no improvement in the patient's oral health. Today, microinvasive dentistry encompasses more economical techniques that impose a therapeutic model based on prevention and the implementation of less mutilating treatments thanks to early diagnosis of lesions using innovative techniques.

The aim of this type of dentistry is to delay a cascade of treatments that will result in major tissue sacrifices, with loss of pulpal vitality and the need for expensive dentures.

In the first part of this paper, we will describe the various elements involved in diagnosing carious lesions at their initial stage, in the context of non-operative caries management.

The second part of this work will present the different ways of managing incipient carious lesions, based on the concept of microinvasive dentistry.

Classification of carious lesions

1. Black's historical classification

This is the first classification of carious lesions on exposed tooth surfaces, proposed by Greene Vardiman Black in the early 1900s.

A century later, this system is still used by the majority of practitioners.

This is a strictly topographical classification of carious lesions (figure1):

> **Class I:** Shaft and fissure caries. This class includes all cavities located in the anatomical depressions of all teeth:
>   - The occlusal grooves of molars and premolars,
>   - The vestibular dimples of the lower molars,
>   - Palatal dimples on upper molars,
>   - The cingulum of the front teeth.
>
> **Class II:** Proximal caries of molars and premolars.
>
> **Class III:** Proximal decay of incisors and canines without involvement of the incisal edges (or angles).
>
> **Class IV:** Proximal decay of incisors and canines with incisal edge involvement.
>
> **Class V:** dental neck caries: a carious lesion located in the cervical third.
>
> **Class VI:** Caries of the incisal edges and cusp tips.

This easy-to-use system is based on a surgical approach to treatment, and does not take into account the severity or extent of the lesions [45].

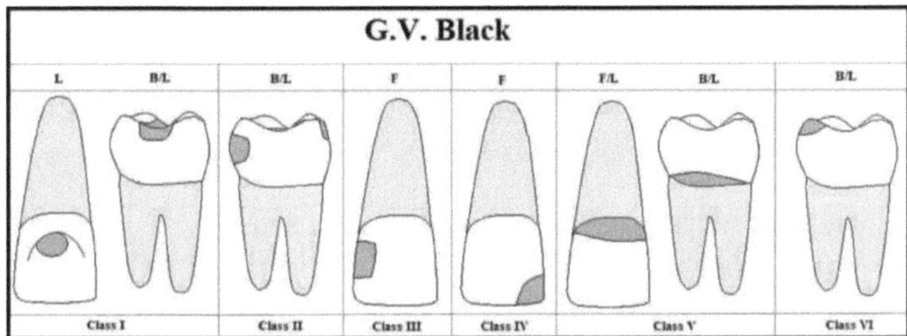

Figure 1: Identifying the classification of carious lesions according to their location [95]

2. ICDAS visual classification

It's a caries detection system, based on visual criteria streamlined in the form of a codified system: ICDAS (International Caries Detection And Assessement System) (Figure 2).

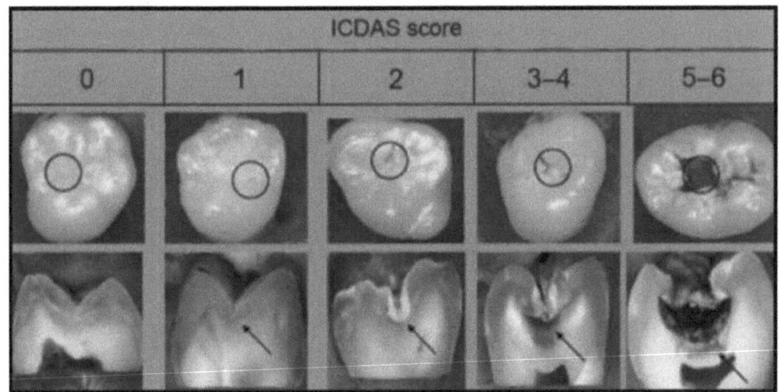

Figure 2: ICDAS clinical visual codes, according to the histological extent of the carious lesioni][71]

Since 2005, there has been a second version of this system, "ICDAS II", which concerns lesions of the smooth and occlusal surfaces. This version is shown in Table I [8].

Table I: ICDAS II classification []8

Code	ICDAS II detection system
0.	Healthy tooth surface

1.	First visual change of enamel 1w (white spot) or 1 b (brown spot)
2.	Distinct visual change of enamel 2w (white) or 2b (brown)
3.	Localized enamel fracture due to decay, with no visible dentine exposure or shaded transparency due to underlying decayed dentine (underlying shadow).
4.	Dark shadows from underlying decayed dentine with or without localized enamel breakage
5.	Distinct cavity with visible dentine
6	Distinct cavity extended to visible dentin

The essential feature of ICDAS is the subdivision of the stages of the dental caries continuum into a variable number of discrete, predictable categories, depending on the histological extent of the carious lesion [71] .

3. Classification by activity

In 2009, Lasfargues and Colon proposed an assessment of the degree of activity of an isolated lesion by assigning it a score based on clinical parameters, previously defined by Erkstanden 2002:

- visual appeal;
- whether the lesion is located in an area that is favourable or unfavourable;
- plaque build-up;
- tactile perception ;
- the condition of the marginal gingiva.

The scores for each parameter are added together. If the total score is greater than 7, the lesion is considered active, whereas if the total score is less than or equal to 7, the lesion is considered inactive (Table II)[46] .

Table II: Evaluation of the degree of activity of an isolated carious lesion [46]

Activity parameter	Degree of severity	Score
Visual appearance	Healthy condition	0
	Opacity (after drying)	1A

	Brown stain (after drying)	1B
	Opacity (without drying)	2A
	Brown stain (without drying)	2B
	Underlined gray shadow	3
	Loss of surface integrity	4
	Punctiform cavity	5
	Extensive cavity	6
Plate accumulation	Unsuitable areas	0
	Favorable areas	6
Sensation at the poll	Smooth enamel, hard dentine	0
	Rough enamel, soft dentine	5
Gingival bleeding on probing	No bleeding	0
	Bleeding	3

It is important for the practitioner to identify the activity of the lesions in order to decide on the treatment to be undertaken: small, inactive lesions require no treatment.

4. Radiological classification

In 1998, Hintze et al. established a scale for assessing proximal lesions according to their estimated depth on retro-coronary radiography. This scale comprises 5 scores (Table III) [1,2].

Table III: Classification by Hintze et al[12]

Score 0	**Healthy tissue (no radiolucency)**
Score 1	Radio-clarity affecting the outer half of the enamel
Score 2	Radio-clarity extending to the inner half of the enamel
Score 3	Radiolucency reaching the outer third of the dentin
Score 4	Radiolucency extending to the inner two-thirds of the dentin

However, this classification system is limited by the difficulty of correlating a radiological image with a histological reality, which can mislead the practitioner.

5. Classification for therapeutic purposes

This is a new classification of carious lesions, established by Mount and Hume in 1997 to compensate for Black's outdated principles. It is defined by three sites (Figure 3), corresponding to areas of plaque-bacterial retention, and four stages, determined by caries extension.

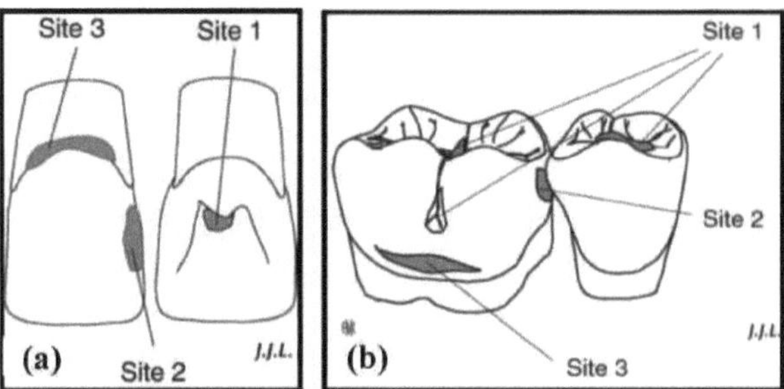

Figure 3: Diagram of cariosusceptibility sites (a) on the front teeth. (b) on posterior teeth[45]

However, this classification only includes carious lesions requiring surgical intervention. As a result, Lasfargues et al. modified the classification by adding a stage 0, corresponding to a lesion that can be treated non-invasively, and presented it in a SISTA concept based on 3 principles:

- principle of tissue economy
- membership principle
- principle of bio-integration [45].

Caries lesions are identified and described in Tables IV and V:

Table IV: The different sites of the carious lesion [45]

Site 1	occlusal lesion: this concerns the cingulums of anterior teeth and the grooves, pits and dimples of posterior teeth.
Site 2	proximal lesion affecting the contact surfaces.
Site 3	lesion originating in the cervix, which may be amelanotic or cementary.

Table V: The different stages of caries lesion development [45]

Stage 0	initial lesion without cavitation, strictly amelitary, not requiring surgical intervention but non-invasive preventive treatment.

Stage 1	lesions with surface micro-cavitations that have progressed to the outer third of the dentine and require restorative treatment as a minimum in addition to preventive treatment.
Stage 2	moderate-sized cavitary lesions that have progressed into the medial third of the dentin without weakening the cuspid structures and requiring minimal restorative filling of the loss of substance.
Stage 3	extensive cavitary lesion that has progressed into the inner third of the dentine to the point of weakening the cusp structures, requiring restorative intervention to fill in and reinforce residual structures.
Stage 4	parapulpal cavitary lesion that has progressed to the point of destroying part of the cusp structures and requiring restorative surgery with partial or total coronary coverage.

Today, tooth decay is no longer seen as a process of continuous, irreversible destruction, but as an alternating phase of demineralization and remineralization. For this reason, in order to ensure appropriate treatment, practitioners must be equipped to diagnose incipient caries lesions (E1, E2, D1) at an early stage. (Figure 4).

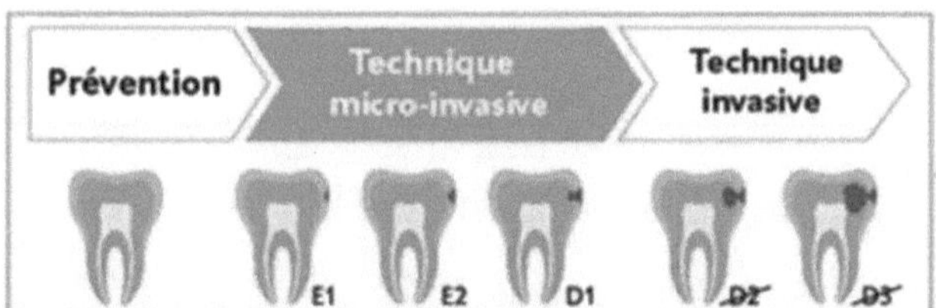

Figure 4: Management adapted to the stage of the carious lesion
E1: ameloid lesion; E2: carious lesion reaching the amelodentinal junction; D1: carious lesion reaching the outer third of dentine; D2: carious lesion reaching the middle third of dentine; D3: carious lesion reaching the inner third of dentine [76].

Diagnosis of initial caries lesions

1. Traditional diagnostic methods

Classically, caries lesions are detected by combining three basic procedures:

- visual examination,
- tactile perception,
- radiography.

1.1. Visual examination

Inspection, according to Ekstrand et al, should be performed on clean, cleaned and dried teeth, in good light and with the aid of a mirror.

Its aim is to detect any opacity, discoloration or change in translucency [12].

However, it is a subjective examination which requires the use of objective criteria to enable several practitioners to interpret the assessment previously established by another practitioner [19], as defined by Corteset al. (Table VI)[12].

Score	Criteria
0	Absence or slight change in enamel translucency after prolonged drying > 5s
1	Opacity or discoloration difficult to see on a wet surface, but clearly visible after drying
2	Opacity or discoloration clearly visible without drying
3	Presence of an enamel cavity in coloured opaque enamel and/or greyish discolouration of underlying dentin
4	Cavity in opaque or discoloured enamel exposing dentin

Table VI: Criteria used during visual examination to diagnose caries[]12

1.2. Tactile perception

1.2.1. Survey

Probing is used to assess the consistency of tooth tissue.

The reliability of this examination depends entirely on the resistance felt by the practitioner. It requires the use of exploratory probes, of different shapes and specific to the sites examined (Figure 5) [12].

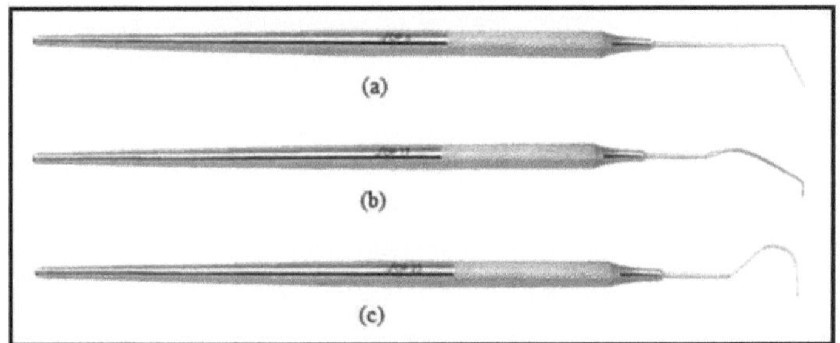

Figure 5: The main exploratory probes:(a) Probe number 6 (b) Probe number 17(c)Probe number 23 [92]

However, probing does not define the degree of activity, extent or limits of the carious lesion. This lack of information allows the practitioner to establish an optimal treatment plan, and runs the risk of over-treatment with significant removal of healthy tissue, without first attempting remineralization treatment[54] .

In recent years, probing has been called into question. The pressure exerted during rigorous probing may produce trauma to enamel surfaces corresponding to sub-surface lesions and the fissure may thus become more susceptible to lesion progression[54] .

In addition, it promotes bacterial transport from one site to another, enabling contamination of healthy sites[12] .

1.2.2. Dental floss

The use of dental floss, described by G.V. Black during his research into cariology and conservative dentistry, will enable the detection of roughness associated with caries damage.

Thus, by pressing the wire against the tooth, followed by vertical movements, it will come into contact with the enamel lesion and fray[88] .

The use of this method in the 19th and early 20th centuries failed to detect early lesions and dentin lesions. As a result, proximal lesions were discovered late and not very effectively. As a result, it cannot be correlated with today's principles of micro-dentistry and early detection[88] .

1.3. Radiography

The precision and orientation of the incident beam make the Retrocoronal or Bitewingle radiograph the reference for early detection of carious lesions, particularly on the proximal surfaces (Figure 6)[1 2].

Nevertheless, this radiography remains limited for initial lesions of the occlusal table due to the superimposition of a large thickness of dental tissue in the vestibular and lingual areas.

On the other hand, at least 30% demineralization is required for caries lesions to be detectable.[46]

According to Lussi, this technique has a sensitivity of 45% on its own and 49% when combined with visual examination for occlusal carious lesions without cavitation[1 2].

According to Vaarkamp et al, at the proximal level, the sensitivity of this technique is between 71% and 100%, specificity between 99% and 100%[12]

.

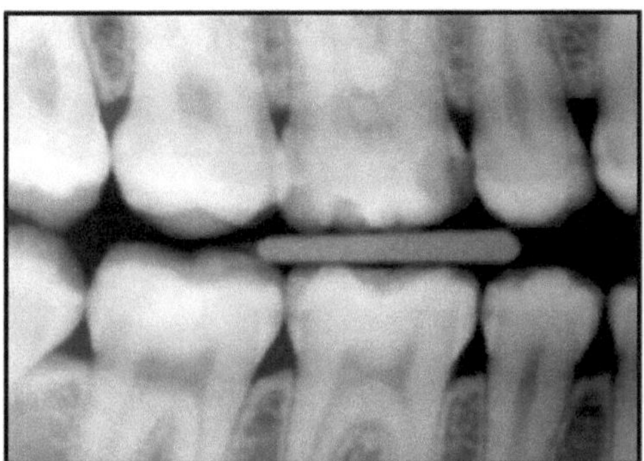

Figure 6: Bitewing radiograph showing: radiolucency score 1 at the mesial level of 6 and 47, score 2 at the mesial level of 15, score 3 at the distal level of 46 and 45.[12]

According to Daudibertiers et al., digital radiography enables better visualization of carious lesions through increased contrast, highlighting of superficial enamel damage, and quantitative assessment of densities by radiometry[12] .

According to Le Denmat et al., the contrast of the observed image can be adjusted to reveal the anatomical details sought by the practitioner if they are contained within the highest or lowest gray level range of the image[12] .

2. Recent diagnostic methods

2.1. Colorants : Caries developers

The possibility of staining decayed dentine using a purplish-red dye, 0.5% basic fuchsin, was demonstrated in the 1970s.

However, this dye is suspected of being carcinogenic and therefore unusable for in vivo caries detection[84] .

Fuchsin has now been replaced by polypropylene glycol-based stains that bind to the denatured collagen present in infected dentin[84] :

- ■ 1% red 52 acid (food red 106 = Rodamine B acid) for Kuraray Caries

    Detector®.

■ blue-black pigments for Snoop®(figure 7).

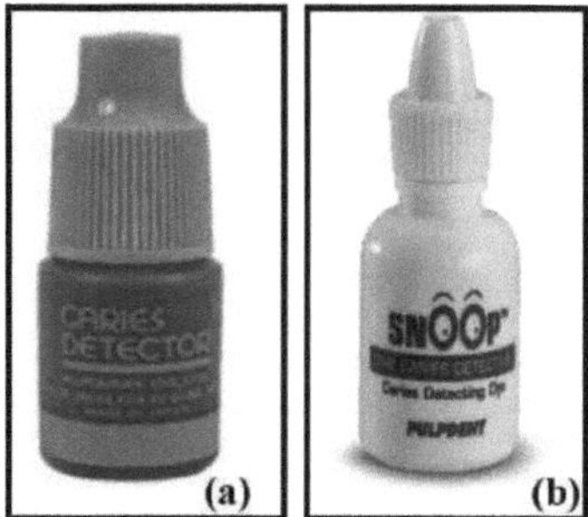

Figure 7: Presentation of dentin stains: (a) Kuraray Caries Detector; (b) Snoop [92]

However, these dyes can lead to misinterpretation on the part of the practitioner:

■ the red coloration may be mistaken for blood from the pulp.

■ blue-black discoloration may be confused with the penetration of metal ions into the dentinal tubules from an amalgam [84].

Demonet's studies showed penetration of *mutans streptococci* and *lactobacilli* beyond the stainable zones. Vaarkamp *et al.* confirmed the limited value of these stains, due to their reduced penetration of the initial lesion[12] .

Thus, when remineralization treatment is planned, the use of these caries developers should be avoided, given the irreversibility of their staining[84].

1.1. Optical aids

1.1.1. Magnifiers and remote magnifiers

1.1.1.1. The magnifying glass

This is the simplest macroscopic optical system.

It consists of a single converging lens and a mount (Figure 8). It allows magnifications of up to x 2, but requires very short working distances, which are not easily compatible with our exercise[52].

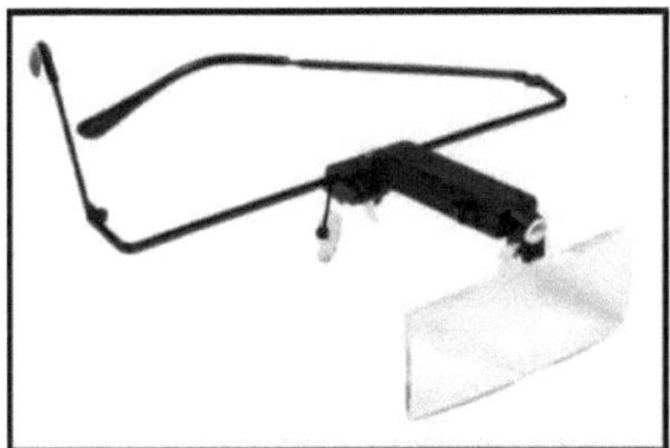
Figure 8: lunettesi mount magnifiers I[62]

1.1.1.2. Remote magnifiers

These are magnifiers combined with a telescope, presented as an alternative to our problem. They offer useful magnifications of between 2.5x and 5x, depending on the fixed focal length of the lens. The latter imposes a depth of field which decreases inversely proportional to the magnification (Table VII)[52].

Table VII: Magnification and depth of field (MALLET, 2002) [52]

Magnification	2,15 x	2,75 x	3,50 x	5x
Depth of field (mm)	23	13.6	11	10.6

There are two types of supports (Figure 9):

- Helmet-mounted remote magnifiers: The helmet supports a remote magnifier, a light source and an optical fiber connected to the remote light generator.

- Spectacle-mounted remote magnifiers: Like helmet-mounted remote magnifiers, these ear- and nose-supported spectacles have the advantage of taking up little space and being lightweight if not fitted with accessories [33].

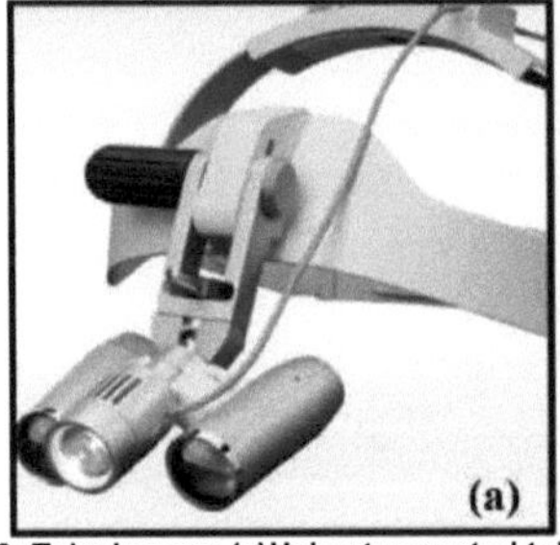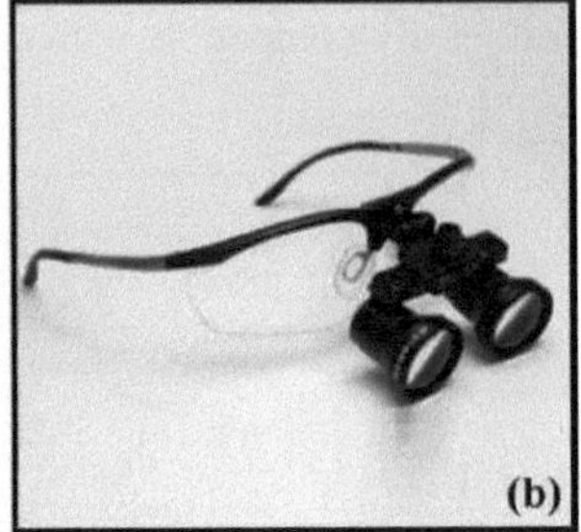

Figure 9: Televiewers: (a)Helmet-mounted televiewers (b)Spectacle-mounted televiewers [52]

1.1.2. The operating microscope

The principle of the operating microscope is based on stereoscopy: i.e., it provides an image to each eye using the binocular head, then by "binocular fusion" provides a perception of relief[52] .

The operating microscope (Figure 10) consists of three parts:

- an optical part,
- a mechanical part comprising the arm and the stand,
- a light source.

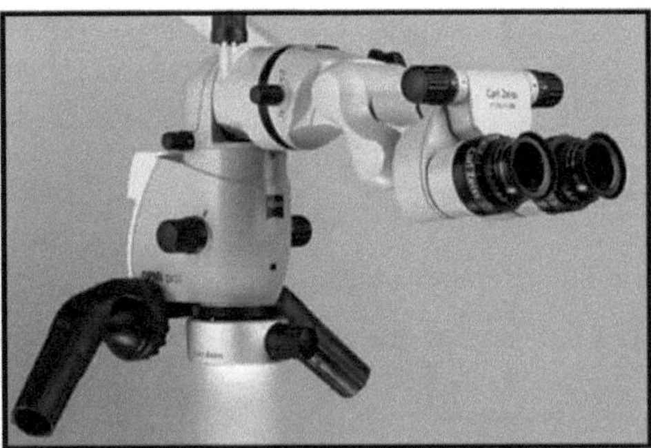

Figure 10: The operating microscope]52

The operating microscope benefits from a considerable depth of field compared to the visual aids described above. This depth of field is adapted to a relatively long working distance, thanks to the increased diameter of the objective. Overall magnification can thus range from 4x to 40x, depending on requirements[52].

2.3. Fiber optic transillumination

2.3.1. Transillumination by single fiber optics or FOTI

The FOTI system uses high-intensity white light, delivered by the fibers of a halogen light source placed at the level of dental surfaces, particularly proximal surfaces [72](Figure 11).

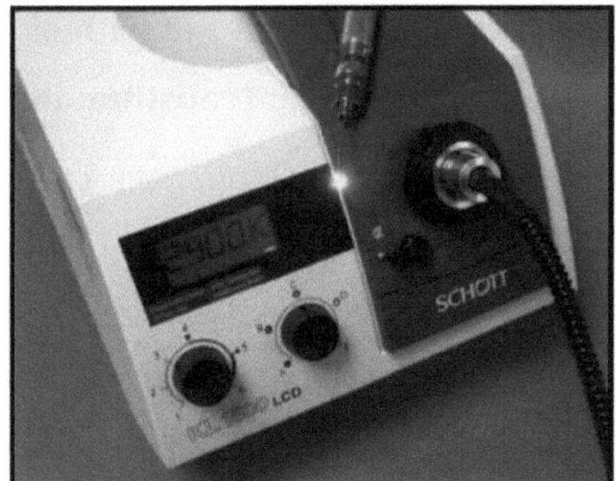

Figure 11: The FOTII device I[72]

Visual inspection of carious lesions is based on the phenomenon of light scattering: when a structural change occurs in the light path, light is diffracted and appears as a shadow in the enamel or dentin (Figure12).

Care must be taken to avoid interference from ambient light, and to watch out for restorations such as composite resins, which modify light dispersion but do not cause carious lesions.

As a result, the examination will depend entirely on the practitioner and his or her visual acuity in detecting these· shadow areas [4 8].

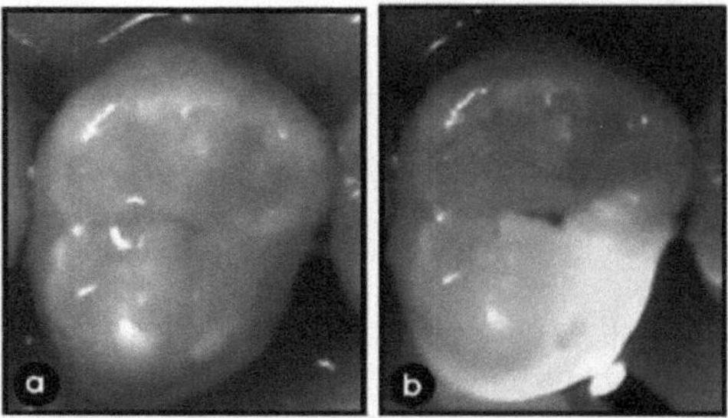

Figure 12: Using the FOTI system: (a)lesion not detected. (b) detection of occlusal caries []72

2.3.2. Fiber optic transillumination with digital imaging or DIFOTI (Digital Fiber Optic Transillumination)

DIFOTI enhances the FOTI system with digitized images for data archiving and tracking over time.

Fiber-optic transillumination was combined with a CCD (charge-coupled device) camera, which are directly integrated into the handpiece (Figure13).

The images of the tooth acquired by the camera are sent to the computer for analysis. The system instantly creates a high-definition digital image of the surface under analysis. The practitioner will be able to study the images through the device's computer screen and look for variations in contrast, helping to considerably reduce the high intra- and inter-examiner variability in diagnosis[72] .

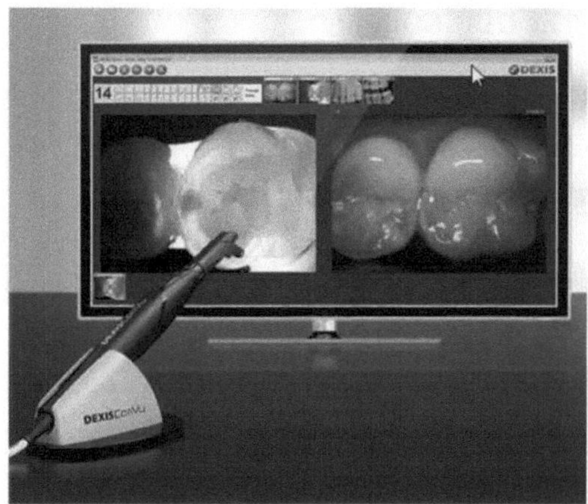

Figure 13: (a) DIFOTI transillumination unit (b) DIFOTI handpiece[ ][62]

The study by Schneider-man et al, revealed the superiority of DIFOTI over radiography in detecting incipient caries, whether on the proximal, occlusal or smooth surfaces (Table VIII)[12].

Table VIII: Sensitivity and specificity values for radiography and DIFOTI in caries diagnosis[12]

	Proximal caries		Occlusal caries		Caries on smooth surfaces	
	Sensitivity	Specific	Sensitivity	Specific	Sensitivity	Specific
Radiography	0,21 à 0,31	0,88 à 0,91	0,18 à 0,20	0,98 à 1,00	0,04 à 0,04	0,96 à 1,00
DIFOTI	0,56 à 0,69	0,73 à 0,76	0,67 à 0,80	0,87	0,41 à 0,43	0,87 à 0,90

2.4. Fluorescence

Fluorescence is the result of the interaction between a wavelength illuminating an object and the molecules of that object. The detection principle is based on the change in physical properties induced by carious lesions [72].

2.4.1. The DIAGNOdent®

DIAGNOdent fluorescence measurement is not referenced by intrinsic changes in enamel structure, but rather by bacterial activity and fluorescence from porphyrin metabolism[72].

Two generations of DIAGNOdent have been marketed.

A first generation in 1998: the **DIAGNOdent 2095** (Figure 14 (a)). The device is connected to a stand on which numerical values are displayed. It comes with a ceramic calibration plate and a flat-tipped insert that detects only caries lesions on occlusal surfaces and smooth surfaces[II*******18].

The second generation: the **DIAGNOdent Pen 2190** (Figure 14 (b)). It differs from the first in that the reading screen is integrated into the device. It is more compact, wireless and weighs just 140g. It comes with two inserts to extend its range of use: a longer, bevelled insert for detecting proximal carious lesions, and a periodontal insert for detecting pockets[18] .

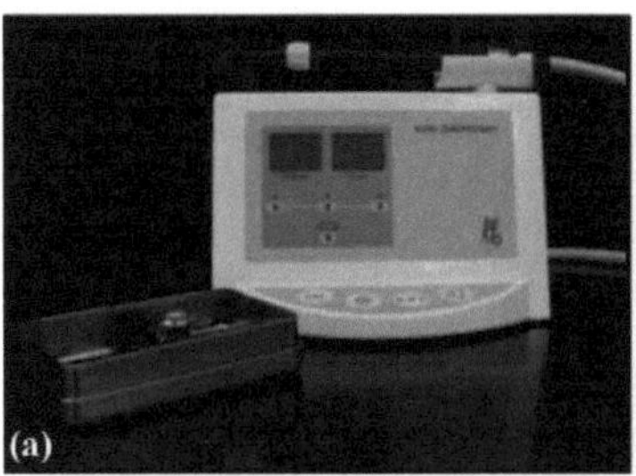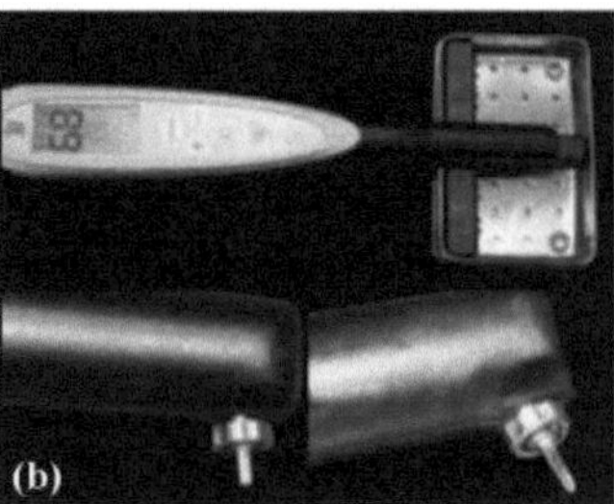

Figure 14: The DIAGNOdent®: (a) DIGNOdent 2095 (b) DIAGNOdent Pen 219QI[1] ≡1

1 consists of a laser diode emitting a power of 1 mW at 655 nm, carried by a central optical fiber. The signal emitted will give a value between 0 and 99, providing information on the degree of demineralization[18] .

Operating protocol :

- Cleaning and drying teeth: an essential prerequisite not only for the system to work properly, but also for a good visual examination.

- Device calibration on ceramic block.

- Measurement of fluorescence on a healthy surface (= reference value).

- The tip is placed on the site to be explored, pointing in all directions so as to record the maximum fluorescence of the demineralization thus examined, in order to avoid missing any significant demineralization.

- The reference value is subtracted from the recorded value to obtain the fluorescence value for the site under examination [28].

The practitioner will establish his diagnosis and treatment plan by comparing the score he has obtained with the limit values provided by the manufacturers (Table IX)[82].

Table IX: DIAGNOpen scores and treatment recommendations[82]

DIAGNOpen score	Level 1	Level 2	Level 3
Occlusal face and smooth surface	0-12	13-24	>25
Histological interpretation	Healthy tissue	Demineralized enamel	Affected dentine
Recommended therapy	Normal prophylactic care	Intensive prophylactic care	Minimally invasive care
Proximal surface	0-7	8-15	>16
Recommended therapy	Normal prophylactic care	Intensive prophylactic care	Minimally invasive care

According to Pretty, evaluations of the device indicate that it may be a promising tool for clinical use: correlation with histological sections of lesions is 0.85; sensitivity and specificity for dentinal lesions are 75% and 96% [72].

However, Bader and Shugars have shown that the DIAGNOdent® tends to find more false positives than traditional methods, and that measurements taken by the device can be distorted in the presence of plaque, calculus, filling materials, food or saliva[6].

Some authors, such as Lussi, have presented treatment recommendations based on the values obtained by the DIAGNOdent.

While others, such as Lasfargues and Colon, do not see this diagnostic method as a primary means of detection, but rather as complementary to traditional means[46].

1.1.3. Quantitative Light Fluorescence (QLF)

The aim of QLF is to determine the fluorescence of the tooth in order to quantify demineralization and the severity of the lesion[18].

The principle consists of using devices to emit violet-blue light with a wavelength between 290-450 nm, such as a silver laser, xenon or LED, which passes through the transparent enamel and excites the fluorophores contained within the amelo-dentinal junction[18] .

Example: The Inspektor Pro® device (Figure 15).

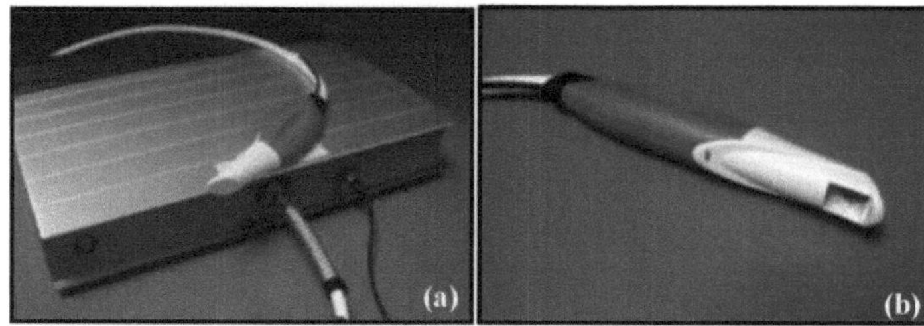

Figure 15: The Inspektor Pro® device (a) QLF unit light box(b) intra-oral camera [72]

The fluorescence process depends on demineralization, but also on remineralization, which leads to an increase in demineralization. Thanks to QLF software and data storage, identical images recorded at different times can be superimposed, enabling us to follow the evolution, stabilization or regression of lesions over time (Figures 16)[72] .

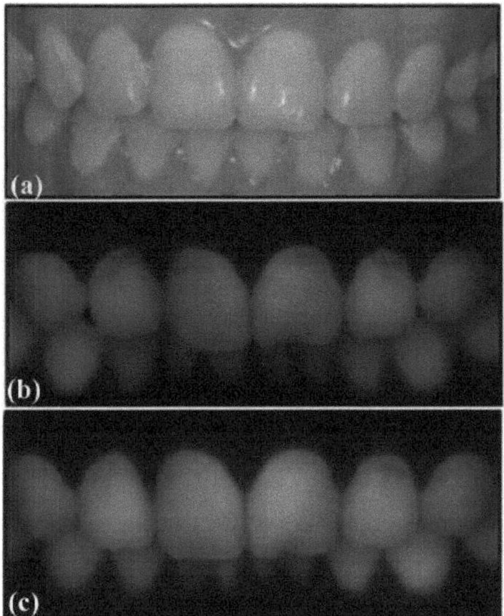

Figure 16: Monitoring the evolution of carious lesions using the QLF system:(a)Carious lesions barely visible to the naked eye. (b)Carious lesions visible by QIF. (c) Disappearance of carious lesions after one month of remineralization by fluoride application[72]

According to Wu et al, there is a linear relationship between the depth of demineralization and the decrease in fluorescence, making this system ideal for detecting initial lesions on smooth vestibular and lingual surfaces, as well as lesions on occlusal surfaces to a depth of 500 microns. However, it is of little use in detecting initial lesions on interproximal surfaces, whose own light-scattering properties can create interference[86] .

According to studies by Alammari et al, sensitivity ranges from 0.56 to 0.74, equivalent to visual examination. However, specificity, at between 0.67 and 0.78, is lower. This prompts us to warn against the risk of over-treatment with QLF[1] .

1.1.4. DELF (Dye-enhanced laser fluorescence)

DELF uses the same principle as QLF, except that it relies on the use of a marker (exogenous fluorescent molecules) to allow detection of the initial

23

lesion, without quantifying the degree of demineralization (Figure 17)[20] .

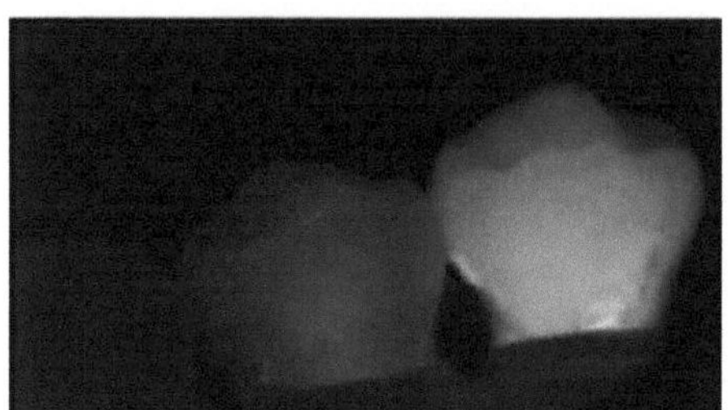

According to an in vitro study by Eggertsson et al., DELF has a sensitivity of 61-79% and a specificity of 86-98%. This is a favorable sensitivity value, approaching that obtained for laser fluorescence (56-74%) and visual examination (58-74%), while specificity is better for DELF and visual examination (8397%) than for laser fluorescence (67-78%)[20] . However, detection artifacts, linked to morphological deviations of the teeth, and dye concentrations in biological structures that are not caries-related, reduce the applicability of DELF in caries diagnosis[20].

1.1.5. Concept Life DT (Laser Induced Fluorescence Evaluation Diagnostic and Treatment)

Intraoral LED cameras are based on the same principle as QLF, but with the aim of illuminating the tooth and producing fluorescent dental images after image processing.

The system therefore relies on the absorption of the incident signal by the porous enamel: the deeper the lesion, the more signal is absorbed.

Thus, the system will highlight healthy tooth areas in green, while carious lesions will appear in red or dark brown [8^2].

Systems on the market :

1.1.5.1. The Soprolife® device

It was launched in 2009 by the French firm Actéon (Figure 18).

The intra-oral camera is equipped with a CCD image sensor and two types of LED that can illuminate tooth surfaces in two modes available to the practitioner:

- Day mode: 4 white LEDs.
- Caries mode: highlights carious lesions in the enamel and dentin via 4 LEDs emitting blue light with a wavelength of 450 nm[82]].

The French firm Acteon has marketed a second camera, called the Soprocare® (Figure18 (b)). This camera features a third clinical mode, the perio mode, which highlights gingival inflammation.

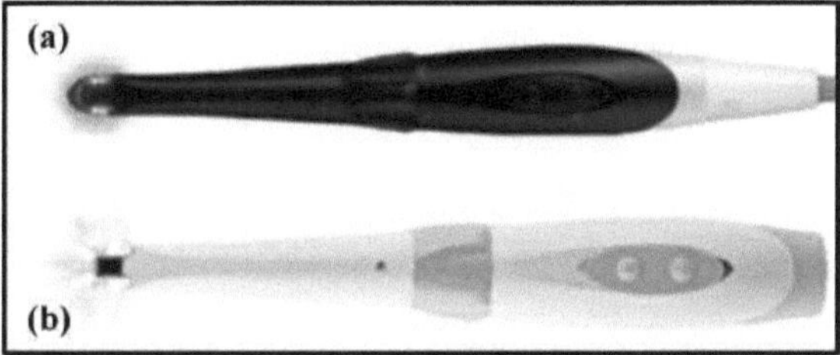

Figure 18: Acteon intra-oral camera(a)Soprolife®. (b) Soprocare®.[82]

Clinical decisions are not linked to numerical values, but to the amplification of visual inspection (Table X)[82] .

Table X: Clinical color guide for LIFEDT and Soprolife®/Soprocare®[82]

Camera. Visual inspection	Healthy dentine	Infected dentine	Affected dentin Active process (light yellow tissue)	Affected dentine Stopped process (brown, very hard tissue)
Soprolife	green	Dark grey	Bright red	Dark red
Soprocare	Grey	Dark grey	Bright red	Dark red

Soproimaging® software enables us to save, compare and modify images, such as on-screen enlargements of between 30 and 100[82] .

2.4.4.2. Operating protocol

Note that these devices do not require calibration with a reference frame.

They are used according to the following protocol:

- Illuminate the tooth in daylight mode and in diagnostic mode at high magnification.

- Note any change in fluorescence of dentin or enamel compared to a healthy area.

- Thoroughly clean the suspect area using pulsed air such as Air-Ngo (Actéon) or Kavoprophy (Kavo).

- Illuminate the tooth again. Any residual red signal indicates the presence of decay or a suspect area (Figure 19)[82] .

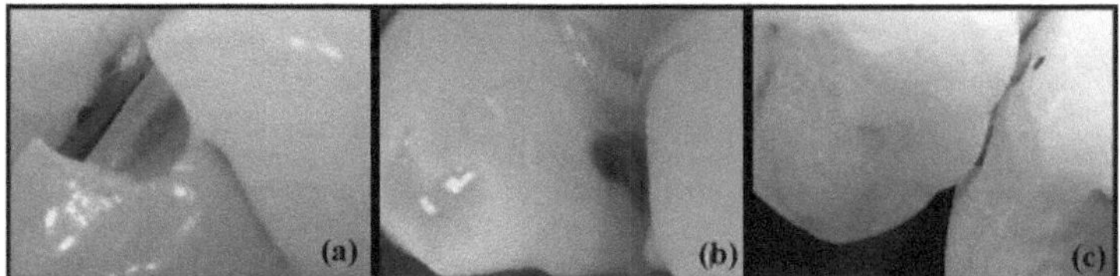

Figure 19: Image obtained with the Soprolife® (a)in full daylight and macro focus mode. (b) in diagnostic mode.(c) after high magnification]]82

1.1.5.2. The VistaCam® camera

This is an intra-oral fluorescence camera marketed by Dürr Dental (Figure 20). It illuminates the teeth with ultraviolet light at a wavelength of 405 Nm and captures the reflected light as a digital image. This filtered light contains the yellow-green fluorescence of healthy teeth, with a peak at 510 Nm, and the red fluorescence of bacterial metabolites, with a peak at 680 Nm[82] .

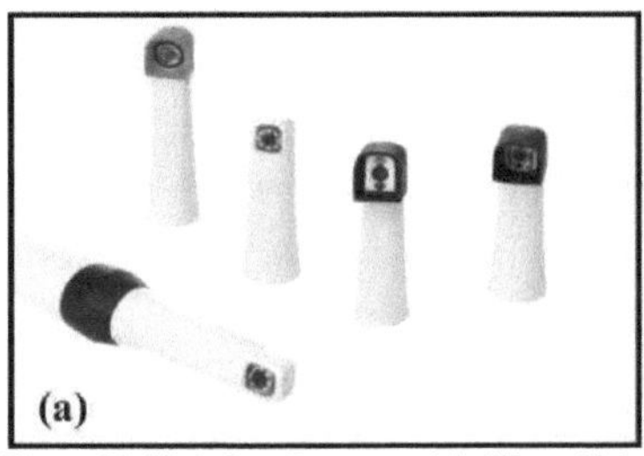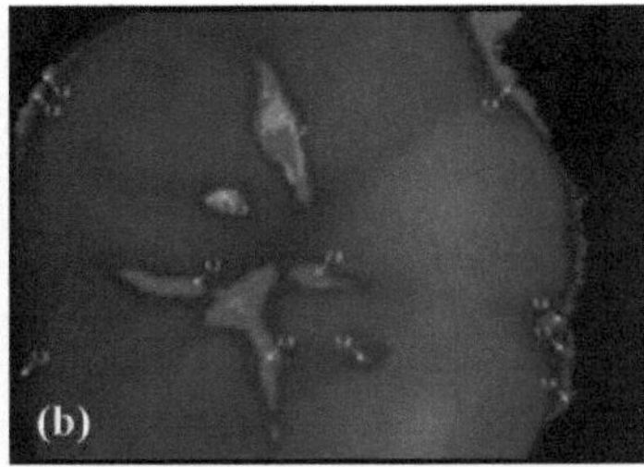

Figure 20: VistaCam® camera: (a) different interchangeable heads. (b)image in fluorescence mode][82]

The software quantifies the green and red component of reflected light on a scale of 0 to 3 with a ratio of red to green, showing areas where the ratio is higher than that of a healthy area (Table XI)[82] .

Table XI:VistaCam® scores and color scales compared to histological reading][82]

Score	0-1	1-1,5	1,5-2	2-2,5	>2,5
Histological interpretation	Healthy email	Initial demineralization of enamel	Deep enamel lesion	Dentine lesion	Deep dentin lesion

1.2. Electrical systems

The principle of these systems is based on electrical impedance, which is defined as the measurement, by means of Ohm's law, of the resistance of biological tissues by sending a low-intensity, high-frequency sinusoidal current through electrodes [82]. The tooth has its own electrical conductance, which is linked to the presence of enamel. In the event of demineralization, the tooth becomes porous and the microcavities are blocked by saliva, which acts as an electrolyte, enabling the transmission of electrical current. As a result, conductance increases and impedance decreases[82] .

According to Jaquot and Fontaine, electrical measurement has a sensitivity of 76% and a specificity of 76% [12].

Devices available in dental practices :

> **Electronic caries monitor (ECM) :**

The ECM device measures the electrical resistance of dental tissue using a single fixed frequency of alternating current. The measurement cycle lasts 5 seconds and is described as a drying profile:

- The tooth must be perfectly clean and isolated from saliva.
- The surface under test, usually a crack, is covered with a conductive liquid.
- The probe, fitted with a coaxial air jet, will sweep over the site, blowing a gentle stream of air to isolate the test site from the rest of the tooth, until a stable measurement is obtained[72] (Figure 21).

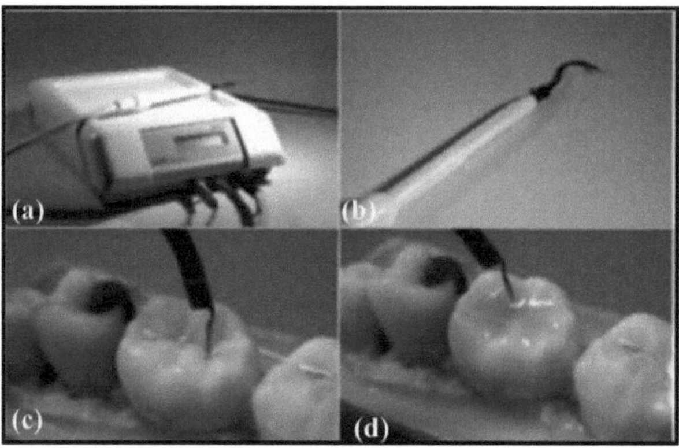

Figure 21: (a) ECM device, (b) ECM handpiece, (c) site-specific (d) measurement technique specific to conductive liquid-coated surfacei[72]

It should be noted that the probe is made up of a multitude of metal filaments, comparable to a brush, which does not allow optimal contact in the proximal zone. As a result, possible measurements will be limited to flat and occlusal surfaces, given the difficulty of implementing the[72] drying protocol. According to Verdonschot et al. ECM does not differentiate hypomeneralized immature enamel from demineralized enamel, resulting in false-positive results in 40% of cases. What's more, it proves ineffective through enamel with high surface mineralization, as is the case in "fluoride syndrome", resulting in false-negatives[35] . Despite these findings, Verdonschot et al. present ECM as a more accurate early diagnostic tool than clinical visual, tactile, radiographic and FOTI examination[35] .

> ### The Carie-San pro® system

The CariScan pro® from IDMoS has been on the market since 2008 (Figure 22).

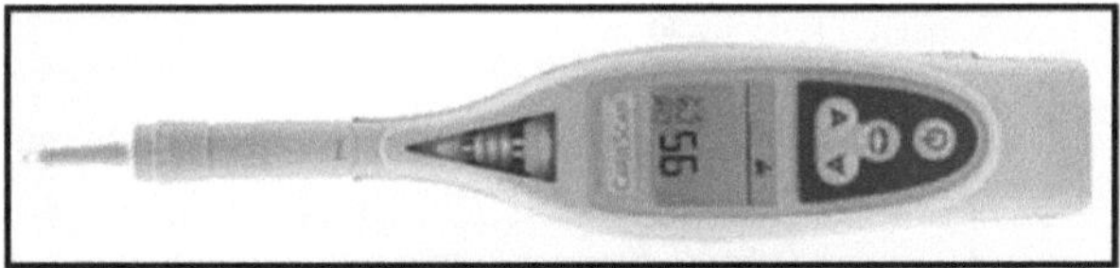

Figure 22: The CarieSan pro®[29]

The principle is based on impedance spectroscopy technology[36] . The system is calibrated at the design stage, and a lip hook is fitted (on the lower lip) to provide a closed electrical circuit. The Carie-Scan pro® will scan several frequencies ranging from 200 to 100,000 Hz and record the data to create a Nyquist diagram for the tooth under test. From this, a tissue resistance value is defined. The M points obtained by measurement are compared with the M points obtained from the Nyquist diagram (Figure 23). The processor analyzes the data and compares it with the system database[29] .

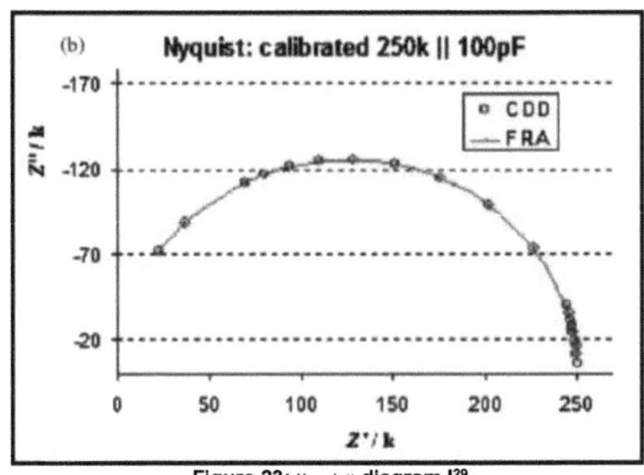

Figure 23: Nyquist diagram [29]

According to the in vivo study by Jablonski-Momen and Klein, the sensitivity/specificity of ICDAS and Carie-Scan were 72.0%/96.6% and

68.0%/90.8% respectively. Comparison of the curves showed no significant difference between these two systems in the diagnosis and detection of dentinal caries on occlusal surfaces[36] .

2.6. The ultrasonic system

> **Ultrasonic Caries Detector®(UCD):**

The Ultrasonic Caries Detector® was developed by Novadent Ltd, Lod, Israel (Figure 24).

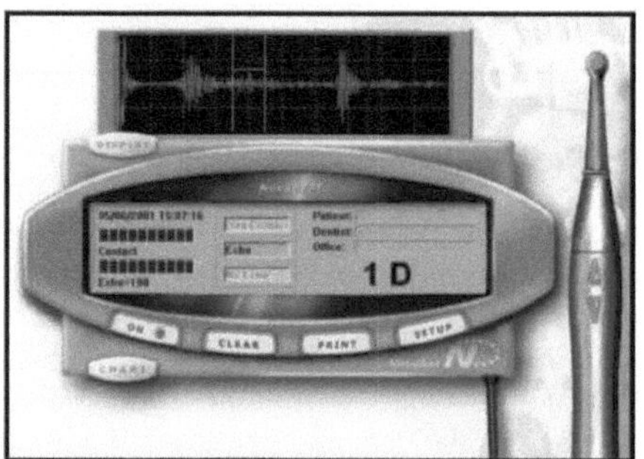

Figure 24: The Ultrasonic Caries Detector®[ ][57]

The principle of this system is based on a beam of high-frequency ultrasonic waves directed at the tooth, which are collected as they are reflected. Each tissue has an acoustic impedance that characterizes its internal sound pattern, whose change can be correlated with a pathological change in that tissue. Thus, the presence or absence of a carious lesion will depend on the dispersion of the waves[57]. In vitro studies by Yanikoglu et al, gave a sensitivity of 88% and a specificity of 86%, superior to that of bite-wing radiography considered the gold standard. In addition, ultrasound was able to detect early "white spot" lesions[87] . However, in vivo studies showed the device to be more sensitive than bite-wing radiography, but less specific: the sensitivity of the ultrasonic caries detector was 0.82 vs. 0.75 for radiography, and the specificity was 0.75 vs. 0.9 .This could be explained by interference caused by saliva in the oral cavity, as well as difficulties in accessing sites during the examination[57]. According to Matalon et al, UCD is a new diagnostic tool that can reduce patient exposure to ionizing radiation and improve caries detection[57] .

Non-invasive management of early caries lesions

1. Remineralization

Remineralization is a dynamic process that promotes the precipitation of calcium phosphate crystals on the surface of calcified dental tissue that has previously undergone demineralization of its mineral component (hydroxyapatite with the formula Ca_{10} $(PO_4)^6$ $(OH)_2$). Under normal circumstances, the demineralization- remineralization pairing constitutes a balanced equilibrium, thanks to the properties of saliva. Saliva, composed of calcium, phosphate and fluoride, restores the tooth's ionic potential. In addition, it has antibacterial and buffering properties that inhibit the acids formed by plaque bacteria [61]. Garcia-godoya reports a critical pH threshold of between 5.3 and 5.7, below which hydrogen ions H+ will react to give hydrogen phosphate of the formula $HPO4^{2-}$, leading to the dissolution of hydroxyapatite[25].

The evolution of a carious lesion depends on several factors summarized in the diagram below (Figure25)[47] .

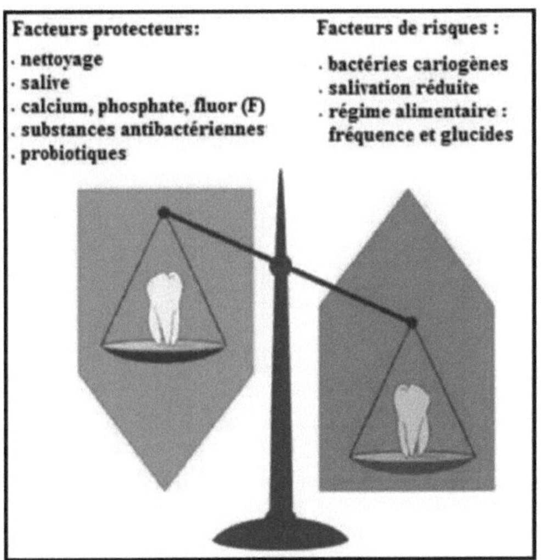

Figure 25: The caries scale[ ][47]

1.1. Remineralization with fluoride

The Sovari and Meurman study, conducted in the 90s, proved the efficacy of fluorides, which inhibited the dissolution of enamel exposed to an acidic drink[79]. In addition, very low fluoride concentrations (below 0.1 ppm) have been reported to inhibit the progression of carious lesions[61]. The use of fluoride has thus become the most effective prophylactic measure for reducing the incidence of carious disease.

1.1.1. Mechanisms of action

Regular topical application loads saliva, dental plaque and oral mucosa with fluoride ions (F-). During the remineralization phase, these fluorides insert themselves into crystals undergoing re-precipitation, helping to form crystals enriched with fluorinated hydroxyapatite. Within crystallites, fluoride ions give them greater stability, and hence greater resistance to acid attack. This explains why demineralized and then remineralized tooth enamel is slightly more resistant to acids than intact tooth enamel (figure 26) [47].

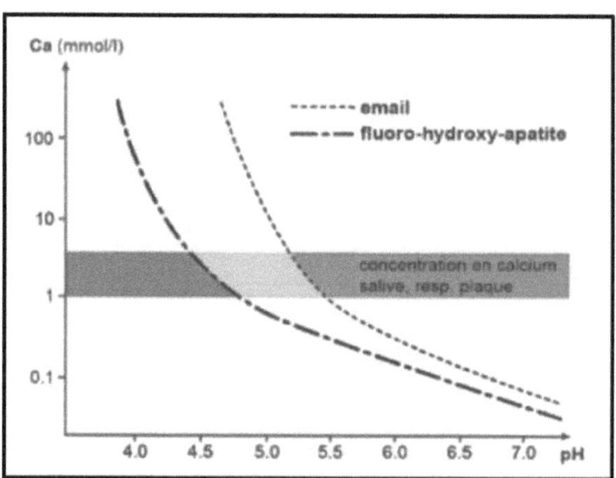

Figure 26: Enamel and fluorohydroxyapatite solubility curves (modified from Lussi 2010)[147]

At higher concentrations, fluoride ions can also precipitate as highly labile microcrystals of calcium fluoride (CaF2), preferentially on demineralized tooth surfaces, but also on healthy tooth surfaces, mucous membranes and within plaque.

The formation of CaF2 constitutes a veritable reservoir of fluorides immediately available when pH falls: these crystals, small granules less than 1 μm in size and relatively stable at neutral pH, dissociate at acid pH, releasing fluoride and calcium ions. Fluorides also have an antibacterial action, reducing the tolerance of cariogenic bacteria to an acidic environment. When the extracellular pH is low, fluoride ions take on the HF form (hydrofluoric acid), which facilitates their penetration into the cell. Subsequently, they dissociate into F- and H+ ions, lowering the intracellular pH and reducing the pH gradient with the exterior, thus counteracting bacterial metabolism.

The main intracellular targets of fluorides are enolase, a glycolysis enzyme, and the proton pump [14].

1.1.2. Sources of fluoride intake

Fluorides occur naturally throughout the world. They are, to some extent, present in all foods and water, so all human beings ingest a certain amount every day.

◆ **Water:**

Fluorine content varies and is dependent on many factors, such as flow velocity, pH, porosity, solubility and rock type.

➢ **Tap water :**

The maximum fluoride content permitted in drinking water has been set by the WHO at 1.5 mg/l [91] .

➢ **Bottled natural mineral waters:**

Fluoride levels vary from brand to brand, ranging from less than 0.1 to 9 mg/l [91] .

The latter are bound by a regulatory obligation on labelling displaying :

■ the words "Fluorinated" or "Fluorurea" or "Contains fluorine" or "Contains fluorides",

■ fluoride content.

■ Suitable for the preparation of infant food", if the concentration is less than or equal to 0.3mg/ml.

■ If the concentration is between 0.3 and 0.5 mg/l, they should mention that supplementation should not be taken.

"Contains more than 1.5 mg/L fluoride: not suitable for infants and children under 7 years of age for regular consumption" if the concentration exceeds the limit proposed by the WHO [9 13,1].

In 2018, Sghaier and Ben Abdallah compared the physico-chemical composition of twenty brands of packaged water marketed in Tunisia. The results of their study showed great variability in fluoride ion content, ranging from 0.19 to 1.77, with an average of 0.64 mg/l[77] .

> **Spring water :**

The limit is identical to that for water from public distribution networks: 1.5 mg/L. In addition, the "suitable for the preparation of infant food" labelling requirements are identical to those for bottled natural mineral water[91] .

◆ **Food :**

Some foods are naturally rich in fluoride. For example:

- Sea fish (1 to 3 mg/100 g)
- Tea (0.5 to 1.5 mg/L) [91]
- Fluoride salt

Salt fluoridation is a Community method used in countries where fluoridation of tap water does not exist. It is authorized in the form of potassium fluoride at 250 mg/kg[91] . Before the age of two, children consume very little salt. Beyond this age, the average dose of fluoride absorbed through fluoridated salt at mealtimes is estimated at around 0.25 mg/d[13] .

◆ **Fluoride topicals:**

Topicals are distinguished according to their use:

> **Fluorinated topicals for individual use :**

- Low-fluoride topicals (<150 mg/100 g or <1,500 ppm):

They generally have the status of cosmetic products and are sold over the counter:

- ✓ fluorinated mouthwashes (200 to 900 ppm): rinse daily or weekly.
- ✓ fluoride toothpastes (1000-1500 ppm): twice-daily brushing [90]
- Topicals with a high fluoride content (>150 mg/100 g or >1,500 ppm): They are

    subject to marketing authorization.
- fluoride gels (1,800 to 13,500 ppm) on the dentist's advice: daily brushing [90]

> **Fluorinated topicals for professional use :**

- fluorinated gels (20,000 ppm): loaded into a mouthpiece which is worn for a few minutes on the chair, once every 6 months.

- fluorinated varnishes (1000 to 56300 ppm): apply once every 4 to 6 months [90].

.

In an in vitro study by Murakami et al. in 2009, 50 human enamel samples were treated with Duraphat® or fluoride gel and then subjected to acid cycles in cola. The results showed that both gel and varnish inhibited enamel erosion in permanent teeth. What's more, during the second phase of the experiment, from 48 hours to 7 days, an increase in hardness was observed[64] .

In Marinho's 2008 systematic review of the literature, the fraction of cavities prevented by fluoride varnish (46%) is higher than those prevented by fluoride gel (28%), fluoride mouthwash (26%) and fluoride toothpaste (24%)[55] .

However, according to the SBU (Swedish Council on Technology Assessment in Health Care), the efficacy of fluoride varnish is not significant compared to that of fluoride toothpaste and mouthwash[90] .

1.1.3. The risks of excessive fluoride intake

The main and most frequent risk associated with excessive ingestion of fluoride is dental fluorosis. The dose not to be exceeded to avoid any risk of fluorosis is 0.05 mg/d per kg of body weight, all intakes combined, without exceeding 1 mg/d (WHO data)[90] . The risk of bone fluorosis is linked to the ingestion of very high doses (10 to 40 mg/d); it has been described in particular in workers in the aluminium industry following chronic exposure to highly fluoridated water (8.5 mg/L)[38] .

1.2. Remineralization with amorphous calcium phosphate casein phosphopeptide (CPP-ACP)

In recent years, a new molecule has taken on a role in remineralizing dental tissue: **amorphous calcium phosphate-casein phosphopeptide (CPP-ACP)**, used under the name Recaldent™ .

1.2.1. Mechanisms of action

CPP-ACP results from the formation of nano-complexes between milk casein phosphopeptides (CPP) and the amorphous form of calcium phosphate (ACP). These complexes accumulate within the plaque, retaining phosphate and calcium ions and creating a strong ionic gradient at this level. Maintaining them on the enamel surface limits demineralization, inhibits cariogenic bacteria and promotes remineralization [73].

1.2.2. Methods of use

The use of Recaldent™ in high concentrations, unlike fluors, is not dangerous. Nevertheless, it should be avoided in patients who are allergic or have a possible allergy to cow's milk casein and/or benzoate preservatives [93].

1.2.2.1. CPP-ACP combined with gum

A recent study by De Oliveira et al. showed that incorporation of CPP-ACP into sugar-free gum, compared with regular sugar-free chewing gum without CPP-ACP and saliva alone without chewing gum, significantly increased remineralization and surface protection of altered enamel [15].

Katakam et al find this association very interesting, as chewing gum increases salivary flow, which will improve the efficacy of CPP-ACP[41] .

1.2.2.2. GC Tooth-Mousse ®

This foam belongs to the MI (Minimum Intervention) range of GC America Inc products (Figure 27) [93].

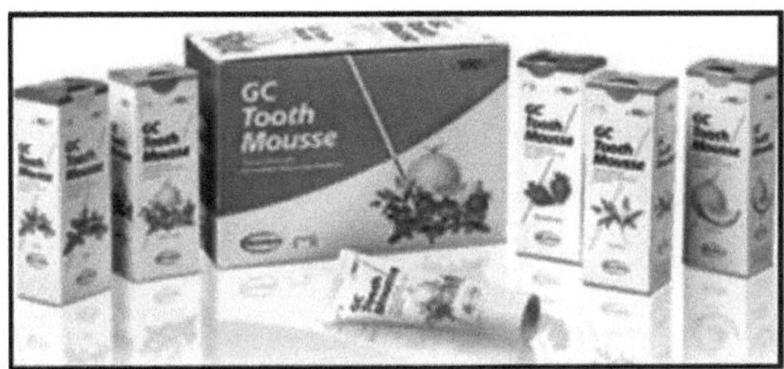

Figure 27: GC Tooth mousse® [ ]93

1.2.2.3. GC MI Paste Plus ®

MI Paste Plus joins the MI (Minimum Intervention) range of GC products. (Figure 28). It combines all the benefits of the revolutionary Recaldent® component in Tooth Mousse with 900ppm of a unique, patented form of fluoride designed for high-risk patients.

This combination results in a CPP-ACPF complex with the ability to supply calcium and phosphate, decrease dissolution and increase remineralization at the enamel surface [67].

According to Jayarajan et al, CPP-ACPF has superior remineralization potential to CPP-ACP [39] . However, this treatment is not recommended for children under 12.

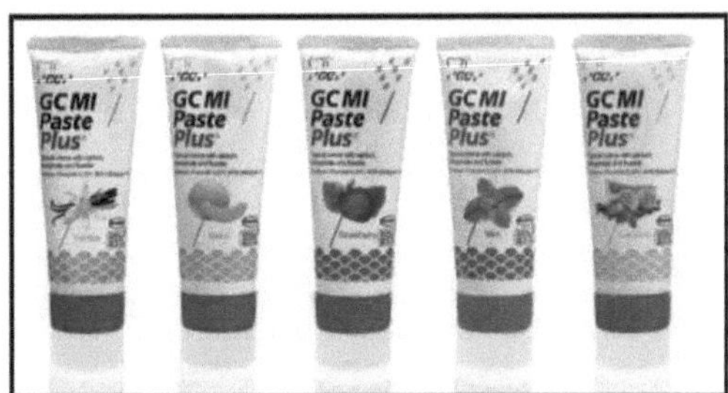

Figure 28: GC MI Paste Plus ® [ ]93

39

2. Ozonotherapy

Ozone (o3) is a naturally occurring gaseous molecule composed of three oxygen atoms. The word ozone comes from the Greek "ozein", meaning smell.

At room temperature, it appears as a pale blue gas with a strong, characteristic odour, similar to that of bleach. It forms our natural protection against the sun's rays, by absorbing the harmful ultraviolet rays present in the spectrum of its light: the famous ozone layer [53].

It has interesting properties in both the medical and dental fields. It is an important antimicrobial agent, often associated with activation of the immune system and improved metabolism and oxygenation of peripheral tissues [65]. Ozone therapy is defined as bio-oxidation therapy, based on a gas mixture of 95 to 99.95% oxygen and 0.05 to 5% pure ozone [53]. In dentistry, there are two ozone generators specially indicated for the minimally invasive treatment of non-cavity carious lesions [53] (Figure 29).

- the Healozone®

- Ozi-cure® .

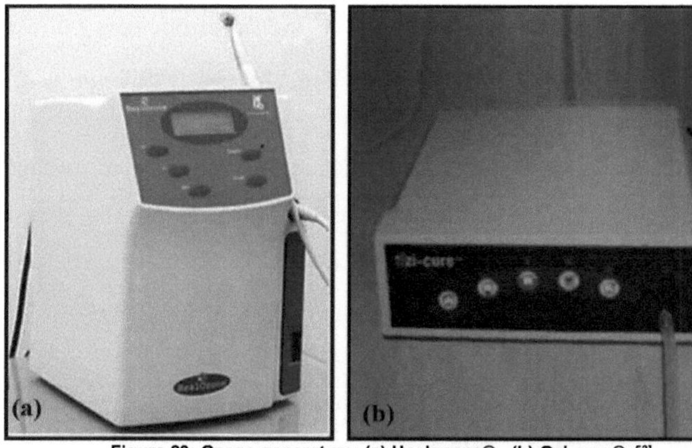
Figure 29: Ozone generators: (a) Healozone® . (b) Ozi-cure® [53]

Millar and Hodson compared the safety of the two systems, recording ozone levels in the patient's nasophryngeal area and near the operator's mouth. They concluded that the Healozone was a safer device than the Ozi-cure. The latter allowed ozone to reach a peak concentration in the pharynx of 1.33 +- 0.52 ppm, which was reduced to 0.22 +- 0.04 ppm when used in conjunction with suctioning. On the other hand, the Healozone showed no leakage, and results were harmful everywhere[60] .

2.1. Mechanism of action

As part of a minimalist approach to dentistry, ozone therapy is painless. It does not require anesthesia, cavities or fillings, making it an alternative to simple milling[53] . Guéders and Geerts have reported reversion and remineralization results ranging from 75 to 99% of early carious lesions without surgical removal, if and only if the operative protocol is followed and repeated at 3 and 6 months[28] .

The management of carious lesions is attributed to ozone's antimicrobial properties, and also to the fact that it oxidizes the pyruvic acid produced by cariogenic bacteria[85] . A concentration of 0.1 ppm is sufficient to inactivate bacteria: ozone disrupts the integrity of the bacterial cell envelope by oxidizing phospholipids and lipoproteins[85] . Indeed, ozone O_3 is a powerful oxidant, its oxidation potential being 1.5 times greater than chloride when used as an antimicrobial agent[92] .

According to Guéders and Geerts, an application of just 5 seconds is capable of eradicating a number of bacteria, viruses and fungi. Generally speaking, ozone is delivered in the form of a 10-second PUFF to eliminate bacteria. A specific remineralization product is then applied to the tooth surface: this is the first step in healing dental tissue[28] .

Huth et al. report on the results of ozone therapy, showing significant improvement over a three-month period[34] .

2.2. Healozone® operating protocol

The time required for application is 25 seconds, during which the cariogenic microflora is eliminated and the healing process of dental tissues is set in motion.

- ◆ **Hermeticity:**

It is essential for triggering the device:

- ■ Place the Cup hermetically on the tooth surface to minimize leakage of ozones, which could be harmful, especially to the patient's lung tissue.
- ■ Once the zone has been sealed, suction keeps the cup in contact with the tooth.

- ◆ **Ozone delivery :**

- ■ An initial PUFF of 10 seconds is applied.
- ■ At the end of this cycle, suction is maintained and a new puff is triggered.

- ◆ **Ozone recovery :**

- ■ Absorption of any ozone residues remaining inside the cup.
- ■ The ozone passes through a catalyst to be transformed into oxygen and

then released into the ambient air.

◆ **Washing with a remineralizing solution:**

■ the device sends a remineralizing reducing liquid into the area to be treated for 5 seconds [28].

Lynch insists on the use of the reducing agent, as it allows minerals to be pumped into demineralized but totally disinfected tissue. This technology must be accompanied by a few instructions to the patient concerning hygiene and diet, such as eliminating or reducing fermentable carbohydrates [28]. However, the efficacy of ozone is disputed by authors such as Lussi et al, who compared the efficacy of ozone with a fluoride gel (Cervitec) in preventing caries lesions in patients with multi-ring appliances. The results showed the development of new white spots to be 3.2% with ozone and only 0.7% with fluoride gel.

As a result, they concluded that the protective effect of fluorinated gel was superior to that of ozone [4³].

3. Erosion-infiltration technique

The concept was developed as a micro-invasive approach to the management of proximal non-cavitating carious lesions, extending from half the enamel to the outer third of the dentin, in order to stabilize them and strengthen the enamel [4].

3.1. Mechanism of action

The technique involves capillary impregnation of the porosities of a non-cavity lesion with a hydrophobic, very low-viscosity, light-curing resin, earning it the name resin micro-infiltration or resin impregnation. This aims to halt the progression of the caries process by obstructing the microporosities that provide diffusion pathways for acids and dissolved materials [17]. In addition, it provides mechanical support to the damaged tissue, reinforcing the demineralized tooth structure. Thus, the barrier created within the lesion will increase the life expectancy of the tooth [59]. Studies by Meyer-Lueckel and Paris have shown that bacteria trapped at the base of lesions can trigger and propagate the caries process. However, in the presence of correct sealing, this process is not described as detrimental, since the number of bacteria in non-cavitating lesions is low[59] .

3.2. ICON® box presentation

DMG offers two types of enclosure (Figure 30):

- a set for infiltration of proximal lesions,

- a set for infiltration of vestibular lesions.

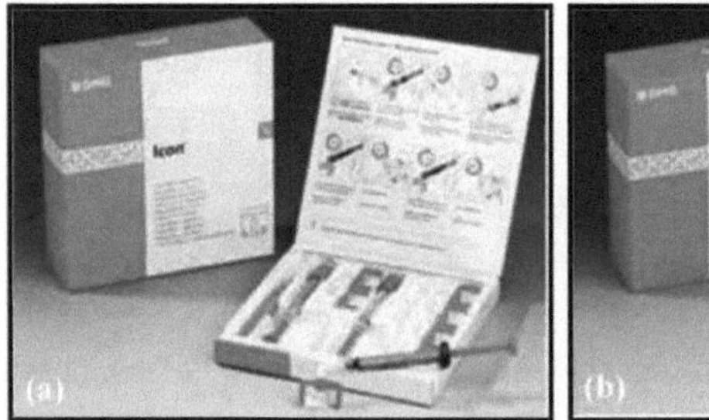
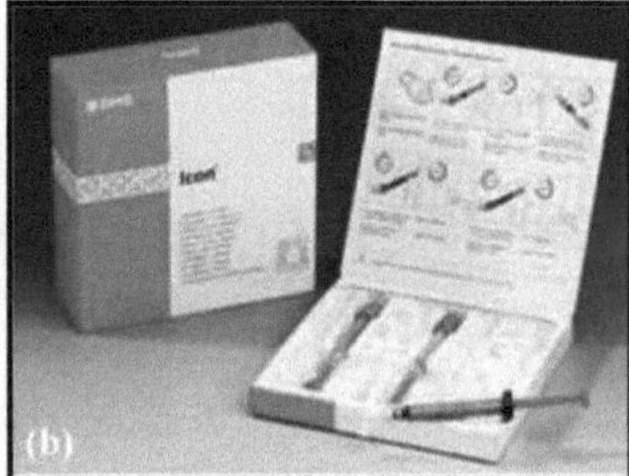

Figure 30: ICON® sets:(a) set for infiltration of proximal lesions. (b) set for infiltration of vestibular lesions [94].

These are differentiated by their applicators (Figure 31):
- Interproximal applicators consist of 2 plastic sheets connected to a 360-degree swivel tip. The sheet on the green side is perforated and will be positioned against the surface to be treated, while the sheet on the white side is impermeable and will automatically be placed against the adjacent tooth to protect it.
- The applicators for the vestibular surfaces consist of a plastic elbow with a foam tip, enabling direct application [94].

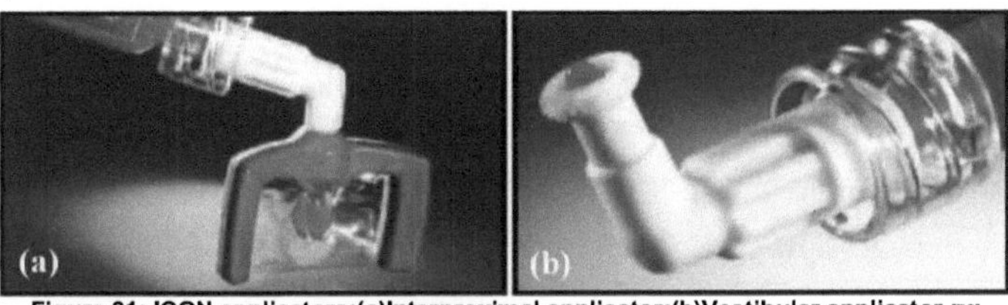

Figure 31: ICON applicators:(a)Interproximal applicator;(b)Vestibular applicator [76]

3.3. ICON® operating protocol

3.3.1. Prerequisites

- Clean the teeth to be treated and those adjacent to them: They must be clean and dry, and free of plaque. We recommend using a brush mounted on a contra-angle.

- Placement of the dam: It protects the gingiva from the risk of lesions associated with the use of hydrochloric acid in the **Icon-etch®**. The manufacturer advises against the use of thermoplastic elastomer-based dams, due to the composition of the infiltrating resin.

- In the case of a proximal lesion, a separating wedge is inserted into the

the interdental space and left in place throughout the treatment[94] (Figure 32).

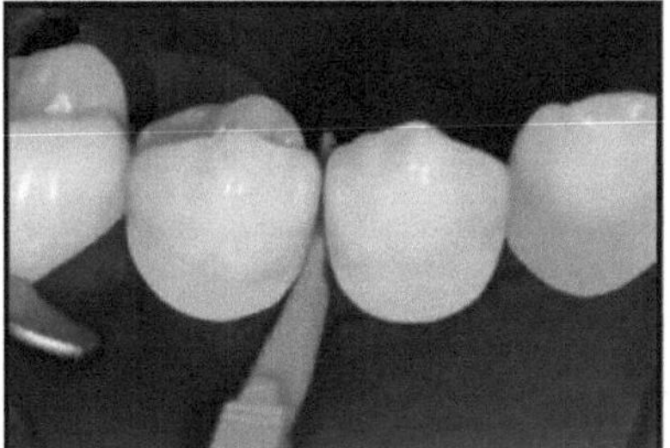

Figure 32: Interdental separation with a dental wedge [94]

3.3.2. Etching

According to Jia et al., the surface layer of natural lesions has greater thickness and mineralization than that of artificial lesions: natural lesions have a thickness of around 40 μm and mineralization of around 83%, compared with 15 to 30 μm and mineralization of 63 to 70% for artificial lesions[40] . As a result, access to the pores for capillary infiltration of the lesion requires perforation or removal of the mineralized layer by etching, using the **Icon-etch®** for 2 minutes (120 seconds), and avoiding the mechanical process, which is uncontrollable in thickness and clogs the pores with debris[4] (Figure 33). On the vestibular surfaces, it is advisable to extend the edges of the lesion by around 2 mm[94] . After aspiration of the etchant, it is recommended to rinse the lesion for at least 30 seconds, followed by drying with non-humidified air[94] . An internal study by DMG© has shown that increasing humidity when using monomer-based resins reduces their homogeneity[76] .

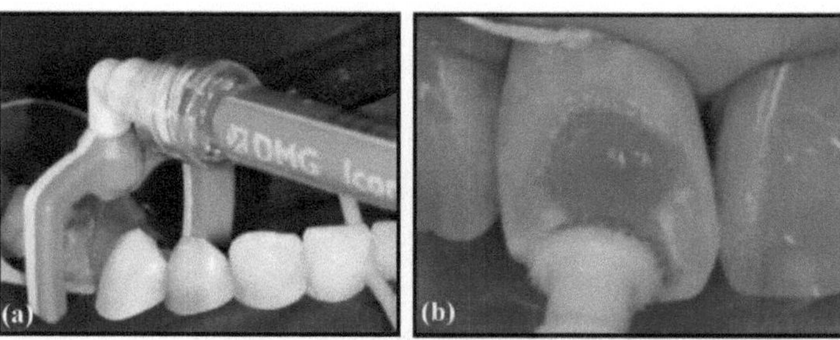

Figure 33: Applying Icon-etch®: (a) etching a proximal surface; (b) etching a **vestibular surface**[94 , 97]

3.3.2. Alcohol drying

This technique is known as "ethanol wet bonding". It involves slowly replacing the water in the demineralized collagen matrix with rising concentrations of ethanol, enabling the latter to penetrate the collagen matrix without causing further narrowing of the inter-fibrillar spaces [4]. This is achieved by applying **Icondry®** to the tooth surface for 30 seconds, followed by air drying [94] (Figure 34). In the vestibular region, **Icon-dry® not** only dries out the lesion, but also enables the appearance of the lesion to be visualized after treatment. In fact, ethanol has an optical effect similar to that of resin, and makes it possible to estimate the result once the lesion has been infiltrated [69]. If there is no change in the appearance of the lesion with ethanol, it is recommended to repeat a 2-minute etching, never exceeding 3 applications[94] .

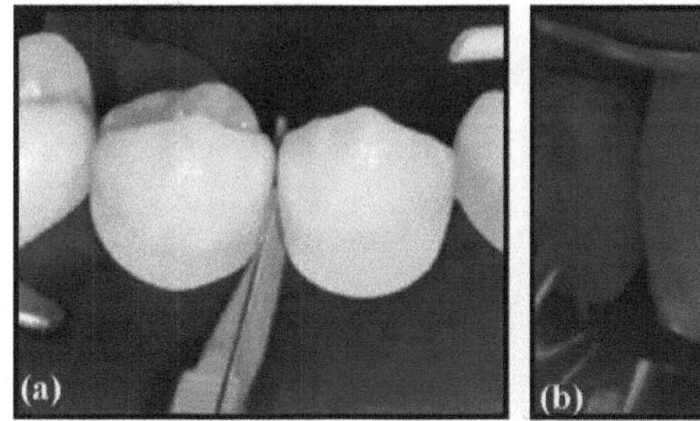
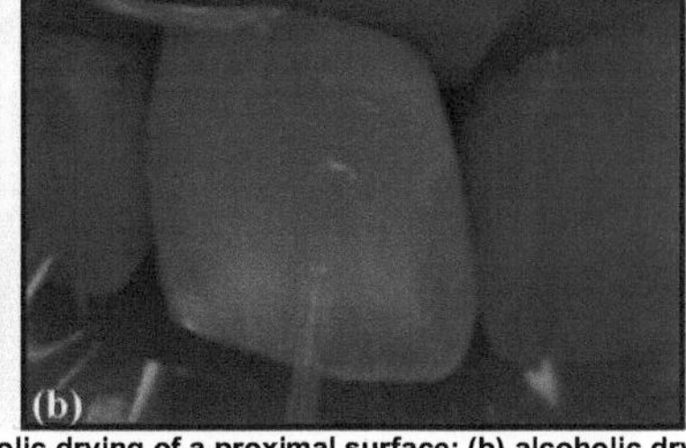

Figure 34: Application of Icon-dry®: (a) alcoholic drying of a proximal surface; (b) alcoholic drying of a vestibular surface [94 ,97]

3.3.3. Infiltration

Infiltration is achieved by a double application of Icon-infiltrant®. First, the product is left in place for approximately 3 minutes, then any excess is removed with a gentle air spray or dental floss in the case of proximal infiltration, followed by 40 seconds of resin polymerization (Figure 35). The manufacturer's recommendations mention an emission value of 450nm with an intensity of $800mW/cm^2$ [94].

In a second step, using a new tip, these steps will be repeated a second time, but with an application time of one minute for Icon- Infiltrant®. This second application is recommended by some authors, such as Paris and Meyerluckel, because of the shrinkage of the material after the first application. In effect, a space will be created and then obstructed by the second infiltration, offering us a gain in surface hardness and an increase in resistance to demineralization, while reducing the risk of creating areas of plaque retention [59].

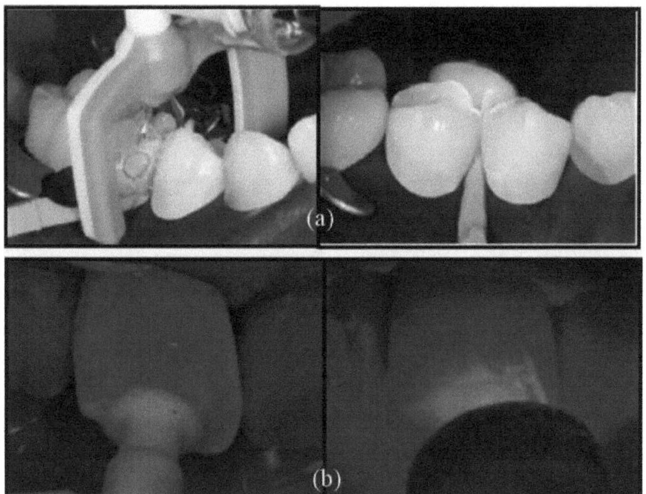

Figure 35: Application of Icon-infiltrant® and polymerization of:(a) a proximal surface;(b) a vestibular surface i[94,97]

3.3.4. Polishing

Polishing treated surfaces will improve the stability of the masking effect.

For this purpose, polishing cups are used on the vestibular surfaces and polishing strips on the proximal surfaces. However, according to Muller et al, the use of polishing strips does not appear to improve surface roughness [63]. Resin infiltration is now considered an asset in the aesthetic treatment of vestibular "cariogenic white spots" thanks to a masking effect that varies according to the depth and activity of the lesion[17] . Azizi explained in his review , that whitish light scattering was caused by the difference in refractive indices between enamel crystals and the medium inside the porosities, noting that healthy enamel has a refractive index (RI) of 1.62 and the microporosities of carious enamel lesions are filled with an aqueous medium (RI 1.33) or air (RI 1.0)[4] . Nowadays, carious lesions are infiltrated with resin (RI 1.52) which, unlike aqueous medium, cannot evaporate and is similar to that of apatite crystals. This makes the difference in refractive index between porosity and enamel negligible. As a result, the lesions lose their whitish opaque color and blend in with the surrounding natural tooth structure[4] . Paris and Meyer-Lueckel reported the first immediate and successful improvement in the aesthetic appearance of white lesions, which remained stable until the 10th month of follow-up (Figure36)[69] .

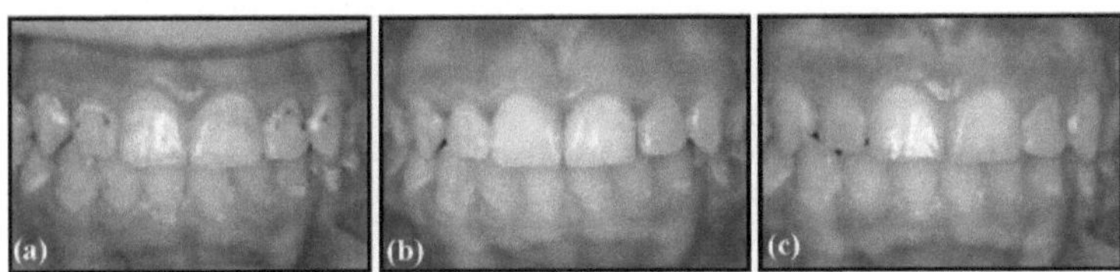

Figure 36: (a) White lesions and brown spots on vestibular surfaces. (b) end-of-treatment result after polishing, (c) result of vestibular infiltration after 10 months. [69]

According to Paris *et al,* the combination of Icon® with preventive measures appears to be an effective solution for limiting the progression of early lesions[59] .

In 2010, a study was carried out on patients with incipient lesions. They were divided into 2 groups: In the test group, lesions were treated with Icon® and covered with fluoride varnish, while in the control group only fluoride varnish was used. After 12 months, a radiological and clinical analysis of the treated teeth showed that the effects of Icon® combined with fluoride varnish were 35% greater than those of the control group. This combination of fluoride varnish and Icon® infiltration resin is therefore an effective method for controlling the progression of lesions on both temporary and permanent teeth[21] .

4. Chemo-mechanical curettage (CMCR)

Today, chemo-mechanical curettage is considered to be a micro-invasive approach to caries removal. The idea of developing a chemo-mechanical curettage agent was first mooted by Goldman in the 1970s. Using sodium hypochlorite (NaOCl) to remove organic compounds from root canals, he noted its ability to dissolve decayed dentine. It was when he tried to minimize the overly corrosive and unstable nature of NaOCl, by incorporating it into Sorensen's buffer solution containing glycine, sodium chloride [NaCl] and sodium hydroxide [NaOH], that he discovered the first CMCR agent and marketed it in 1972 under the name GK- 101[37] . In 1984, following several stages of improvement, the Caridex system obtained US FDA (Food and Drug Administration) approval, but for practical reasons its use remained very limited[56] . Currently, 2 new systems have been introduced to the market:

- Carisolv® in 1998
- Papacarie® - in 2003

Their principle is to apply a gel, which acts selectively on the decayed tissue, softening the infected dentine while preserving the affected dentine, and then remove it using an excavator or specific instruments[37] .

4.1. The Carisolv® system

4.1.1. Presentation

It was launched in 1998 by Medi Team, Sweden.

The system consists of two gels, and takes the form of a double-compartment syringe fitted with single-use mixing tips (Figure 37):

- The first compartment contains 2.5ml of uncolored multimix gel, a mixture of 3 amino acids: leucine, lysine and glutamic acid, plus sodium hydroxide, sodium chloride and carboxymethyl cellulose.

- the second compartment contains 0.95% sodium hypochlorite at a rate of 2.5ml[58] .

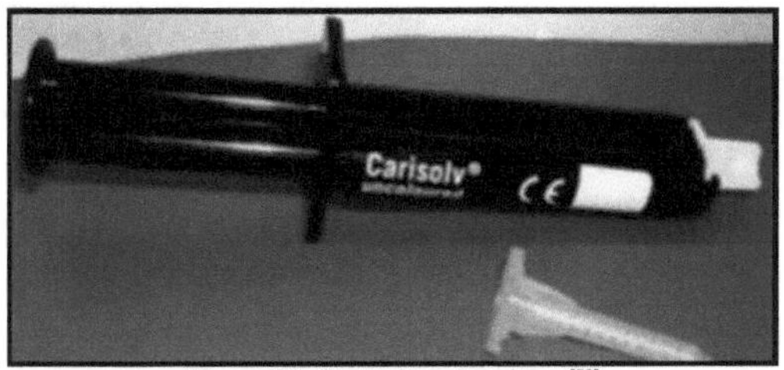
Figure 37: Carisolv gel syringe [58]

Once mixed, the gel is colorless, preventing secondary discoloration of residual tissue prior to the obturation phase. On the other hand, the reduced viscosity of the gel hinders placement[58] .

4.1.2. The mechanism of action

The mode of action is a dissolution of collagen altered by the carious process. The three amino acids undergo chlorination by the highly active ClO- ion of sodium Lhypochlorite. This chlorination reduces the deleterious activity of Lhypochlorite on healthy tissue, while allowing the chloro-amino acids to take effect. Once modified, these amino acids act on the hydrogen bonds and other forces stabilizing the triple helix of affected collagen, without disrupting healthy covalent bonds. The modified affected collagen is then removed using specific hand instruments (Figure 38), depending on the site and stage of decay, thus avoiding the need for milling[83] .

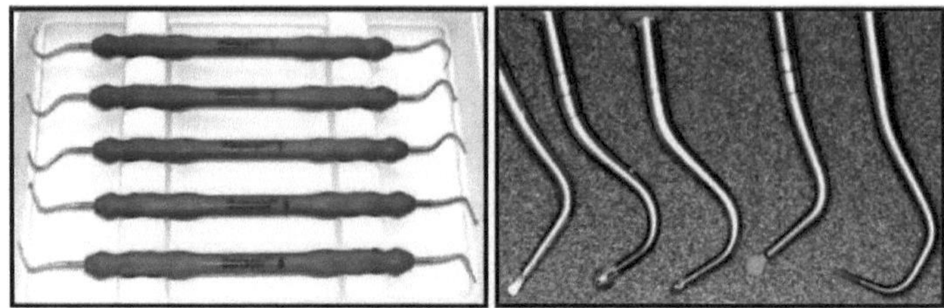

Figure 38: Carisolv instrumentation [58]

4.1.2. Operating protocol

- The gel is deposited in contact with decayed dentine using a double-mix syringe fitted with a disposable applicator tip.

- This is stirred with a *Carisolv®* instrument to accelerate the chemical reaction.

- It is left in place for 30 seconds.

- Then, using specific instruments, dentine will be scraped rather than excavated. This will reduce wear and maintenance.

- This sequence is repeated until the gel is no longer cloudy: this indicates complete elimination of decay.

- Finally, remove any remaining gel with moistened cotton balls, then rinse and dry the cavity [58].

Clinical application of the *Carisolv®* system on a 28-year-old patient (Figure 39).

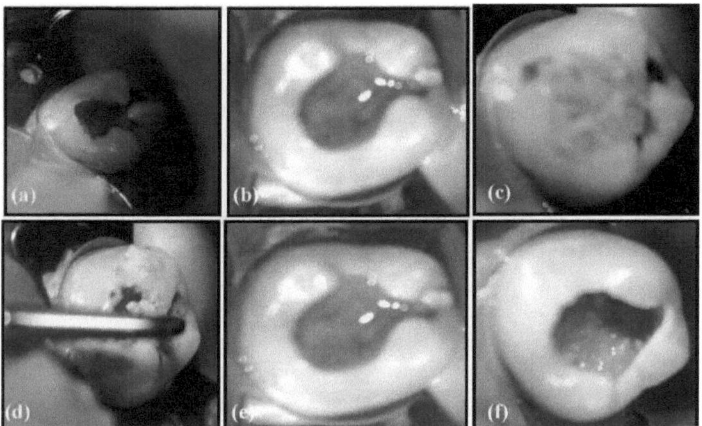

Figure 39: (a) Caries Site1/Stage 3 on 37.(b) Gel applied for 30 seconds;(c) Gel clouded (d)Infected dentin scraped (e) Gel renewed;(f) Dentine curettage completed [58].

Referring to the meta-analysis carried out by Maru et al in 2015, based on 26 studies, comparing the Carisolv system with traditional milling techniques: the results showed that Carisolv took longer (8.65 ± 0.09 and 8.97 ± 0.66 min) than the rotary milling method (3.65 ± 0.05 and 4.09 ± 0.29 min). However, it had the advantage of reduced pain (14.67 for Carisolv vs. 6.76 for rotary milling), less need for anesthesia (1.59% vs. 10.52%). Thus, despite longer treatment times, the procedure was readily accepted and preferred by adults, and even more so by children (18.68% vs. 4.69%)[56] . The 2004 study by Azrak et al, comparing the Carisolv system's reduction in cariogenic flora with that of conventional excavation, was carried out on 21 children (mean age 43.5 +/- 12 months) with 42 carious lesions of comparable degrees of destruction. Samples of decayed dentine were taken with a sterile scraping instrument, before and after removal of all softened dentine. After 24 h incubation, 12% of decayed dentin samples contained more than 10^6 bacteria, 23.8% contained more than 10^5 lactobacilli. The results of both caries removal methods resulted in a statistically significant reduction of ($P = 0 - 0001$), in at least 90.5% of samples taken after removal.

53

The total number of bacteria was below 10^2 and in 95.2% of cases, lactobacilli fell below 10^2 . This shows that chemo-mechanical curettage in children using Carisolv is as effective as conventional methods. It can therefore be considered a suitable alternative[5] .

4.2. The Papacarie ® system

4.2.1. Presentation

Papacarie, which means "eating cavities", is a gel that was introduced in Brazil in 2003, after being patented, registered and approved by ANVISA (Agence National de Vigilance Sanitaire)[37] (Figure 40).

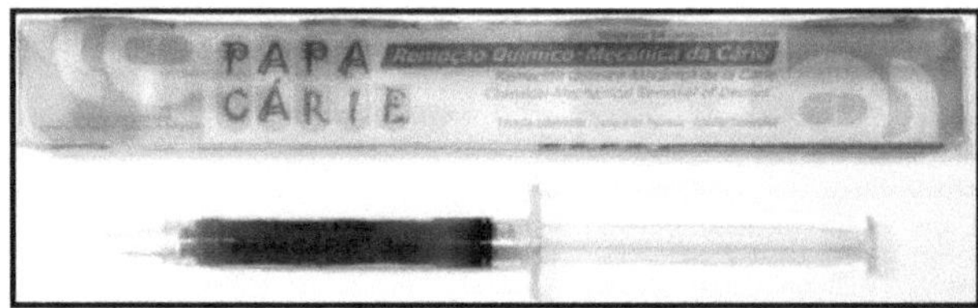

Figure 40: Papacarie 1[37

Its main components are :

◆ **Papain:**

It is a bactericidal proteolytic enzyme with a bacteriostatic effect. It is considered a debriding anti-inflammatory that does not damage healthy tissue and accelerates the scarring process [37].

◆ **Chloramines:**

These are amines containing at least one chlorine atom, which is directly bonded to nitrogen atoms. They have bactericidal and disinfectant properties. They also affect the structure of collagen by disrupting the hydrogen bond, thus facilitating the removal of decayed tissue[37] .

◆ **Blue toluidine:**

It is a photosensitive pigment that binds to the bacterial membrane[37] .

4.2.2. Mechanism of action

Infected tissue lacks a plasma anti-protease called anti-trypsin. The latter inhibits protein digestion in healthy tissue. Its absence will therefore enable papain to break down the partially degraded collagen in infected dentine, while sparing the affected dentine [37].

4.2.3. Operating protocol

The carious lesion is covered by Papacarie gel, without disturbing it, for 30 s and between 40-60 s if the carious process is chronic. Following collagen degradation :

- oxygen will be released, causing bubbles to appear on the surface.
- the gel becomes cloudy.

These signs show that the elimination process can begin.

- Scrape gently and without pressure, using pendulum-like movements with an excavating spoon.
- The gel is reapplied to the excavation site until it is no longer cloudy.
- Remove gel and wipe cavity with damp absorbent cotton, then rinse.
- Complete removal of carious tissue is characterized by the vitreous appearance of the cavity [37].

Singh et al 2011, evaluated and compared the antimicrobial efficacy, time consumption efficacy, as well as pain perception, of the chemo-mechanical caries removal agent Papacarie® and the conventional method. Their study involved forty children (aged 4 to 8) with 2 carious lesions with comparable degrees of destruction. The results were as follows:

- The time spent using chemo-mechanical means (328.5 ± 45.26 s) was 3 times longer than the time spent using the conventional method (124.6 ± 22.76 s) ($p < 0.01$).
- The pain score during the chemomechanical caries removal method

was 1.525 versus 6.65 when the conventional method was used (p <0.01)[78] .

- As for their bacteriological effectiveness:

The average total viable number of S. viridians was 3.575 bacteria / ml before treatment and was reduced to 0.675 after caries removal with the chemo-mechanical agent and to 0.425 with the conventional method.

The difference between the pre-treatment sample score and the post-treatment sample score was statistically significant in both groups (p <0.01). This corresponds to an average reduction in the total viable number of 87.94% and 81.12% for the conventional and chemo-mechanical methods, respectively[78] .

In 2016, based on bacteria counts, Muna et al recomparison the bacteriological efficiencies of Papacarie gel and conventional methods.

The results showed a significant reduction in the average bacterial counts, taken from caries cavities, from (4300.33) to (285.33) for treatments with Papcarie gel and from (4425.67) to (411.33) for conventional treatment[2] .

5. ART (atraumatic restorative treatment)

Atraumatic restorative treatment is an entirely manual procedure, suitable for carious lesions that do not extend beyond the outer third of dentine. It has been defined by Frencken and Van Amerongen as follows:

"ART is a *minimally* invasive approach to both prevent the onset of carious lesions and halt their progression. It comprises two elements: the reconstitution of cavitated dentinal lesions and the sealing of adjacent at-risk pits and fissures. ART restoration involves the removal of softened, completely demineralized decayed tooth tissue using hand instruments. This is followed by restoration of the cavity with an adhesive dental material, simultaneously sealing any remaining at-risk fissures. ART sealing involves the application of high-viscosity glass ionomer cement (CVI) into the pits and fissures under digital pressure." [32].

ART was originally developed in the mid-80s as an effective response to the need for preventive and restorative care among disadvantaged social groups in poorer countries. But the fact that, in this treatment, recourse to anesthesia is very rare, has broadened its indications in wealthier countries, as an approach of choice for children, phobic patients and certain anxious adults [32].

The ART protocol is not dependent on electricity or a dental practice. It can be used in facilities such as schools, psychiatric hospitals or retirement homes[32] .

5.3. Instrumentation

The instruments needed to implement ART [32].

- **A basic tray:** probe, mirror, scoop.

- **A small enamel chisel:** provides access to softened dentine (Figure 41(a)).

- **2 excavators :**

✓ Of different sizes, a small one with a working part about 1 mm in diameter, and a slightly larger one used to remove softened dentine (Figure 41 (b)).

✓ The larger excavator can also be used to place restorative material under the enamel and to remove excess material.

- A small filling and shaping spatula ("Ash 6 special" type): to apply CVI and remove excess material (Figure 41 (c)).

- A special instrument, the Enamel Access Gutter, has two active pyramid-shaped ends:

✓ The largest can be used when the cavity opening is relatively large, but still needs to be enlarged.

✓ The smaller one is used for small cavities where it is difficult to use the enamel chisel (Figure 41 (d)).

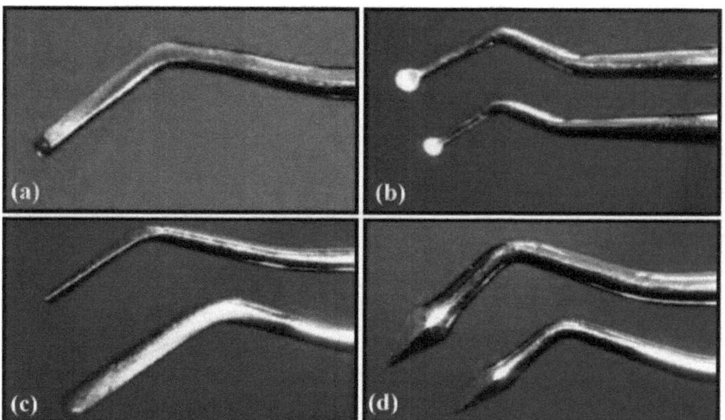

Figure 41: ART instruments: (a) Enamel chisel (b) Excavators (c) Ash 6 special spatula (d) Enamel Access Cutter (EAC) [32]

5.2. Equipment and materials

■ Usual dental office consumables: e.g. cotton rolls, Vaseline, etc.

■ A CVI validated for ART use (HVGIC): a high viscosity, high strength CVI such as: Fuji IX™ CVI (GC International), Ketac™ Molar, Ketac™, Easymix (3M ESPE), Chemflex™ (Dentsply)[32] .

5.4. Operating protocol

Preparation of ART instruments and materials prior to the clinical procedure. Isolation of the surgical site. [32]

For ART, cotton rolls are sufficient, although all bonding protocols recommend the use of a dam, as contamination of the operative site with saliva or blood will affect the bonding of the CVI to the tooth surface.

◆ **Examination of the decayed tooth[32] :**

■ Carefully remove all food debris and/or plaque from wells and grooves using a pressureless probe.

- Clean the tooth surface with a cotton pellet soaked in water, then dry with a dry pellet.

❖ **Establishing access proportional to the carious lesion[32] :**

Generally, an enamel chisel is used to widen the entrance to access deeper areas (Figure 43). Back and forth rotation will fracture the fragile, demineralized enamel surrounding the cavity and allow adequate access to the decayed dentin for the smallest excavator. If the carious lesion is very small compared to the enamel chisel, the small active end of the Enamel Access Cutter (EAC) can be used to fracture the less resistant demineralized enamel and increase access. It should be noted that the EAC must not be used to create iatrogenic cavities. In case of doubt, it is safer to place a therapeutic sealant directly, without any special preparation.

❖ **Curettage of softened dentine:**

Unsupported enamel will only be removed if additional access is required to remove the entire JAD-softened dentin. It will be partially and gently fractured with the blade of the enamel chisel in the direction of the enamel prisms (Figure 42). In cases where the enamel is too thin and brittle, but does not prevent the softened dentin from being curetted, it will be left in place as it will become supported once the cavity is restored with CVI.

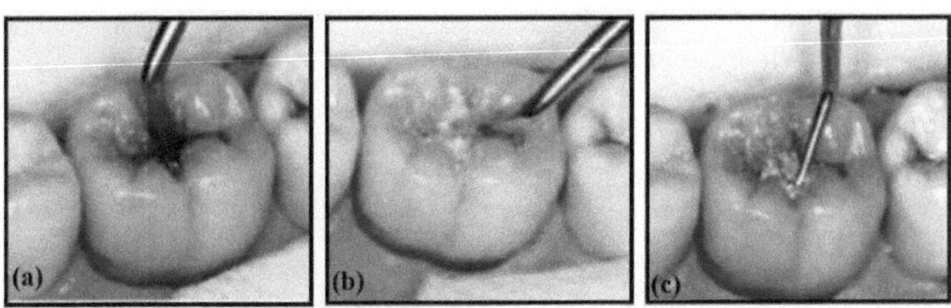

Figure 42: Excavation of crimped tissue by ART. (a) Enamel chisel in place;(b) Access made with the cutting edge of the enamel chisel. (c) Curettage of softened dentin. [32]

◆ **Conditioning of the cavity, shafts and adjacent grooves:**

It should be noted that the use of manual instruments produces a dentin sludge that should be removed with a dentin conditioner to improve the chemical and mechanical bonding of the CVI to dental tissues[32] .

◆ **CVI mix :**

Accurate mixing of the CVI is essential for reliable results.

◆ **Cavity sealing and filling of wells and grooves:**

Using the round part of the excavator or the small filling and shaping spatula, we will :

- Insert the CVI quickly into the lesion, as long as its surface is shiny, so as not to alter its bonding properties.

- Avoid air bubbles, by compacting the CVI under the enamel overhangs before filling the core cavity.

- Fill the slightly excess cavity, then all wells and grooves adjacent to the cavity (Figure 43).

Next, the excess CVI is moved to the outer edges of the occlusal surface, using the "Press Finger" technique (Figure 43). Finally, the excess CVI is removed with the obturation spatula or larger-gauge excavator, taking care not to disinsert the restoration (Figure 43).

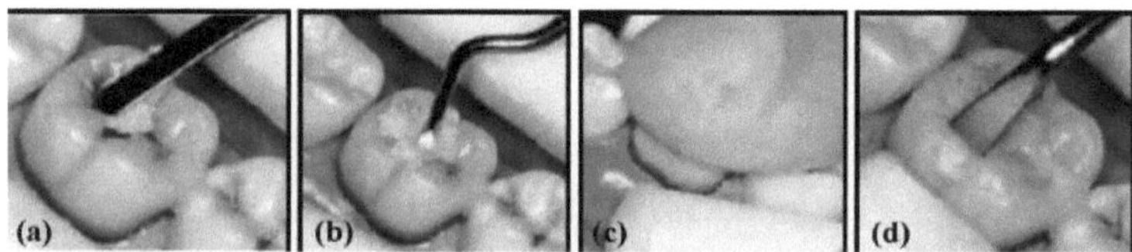

Figure 43: Filling the cavity with CVI; (a) Inserting the CVI with the rounded part of the spatula; (b) Spreading excess CVI over the network of wells and grooves adjacent to the cavity; (c) Moving the CVI using the digital pressure technique;(d) Removing excess CVI with the Ash 6 special. [3 2]

- Check the occlusion before the material sets completely.
- Vaseline the filling or cover it with a varnish
- Advise patient not to eat for at least one hour.

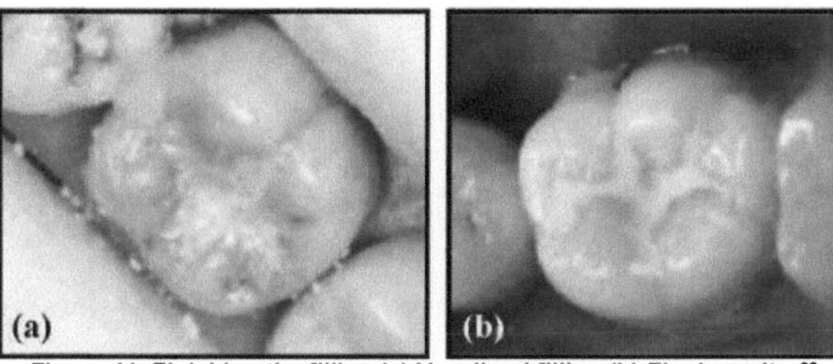

Figure 44: Finishing the filling (a) Vaselined filling (b) Final result [ ]32

According to the 2017 meta-analysis by Frencken et al, the weighted mean survival of ART / HVGIC sealants after 1, 2, 3, 4, 5 and 6 years was 79%, 69%, 68%, 62%, 63% and 59% respectively. The effect of ART / HVGIC sealants in preventing cavitary dentine lesions appears to be very high: the weighted average of cavitary dentine lesions in sealed pits and fissures after 1, 2, 3, 4, 5 and 6 years was 0.4%, 2.4%, 2.8%, 4.1%, 9.6% and 15% respectively[24] .

6. Microdentistry burs

The use of traditional burs in modern dentistry is no longer in vogue. They don't care about keeping enamel unsupported, and their use has revealed a significant iatrogenic effect on the dentin-pulp complex. What's more, the results of their preparations are no longer in line with the requirements of microinvasive preparations. As a result, new burs have been developed [66].

5.5. Micro strawberries

These micro burs are designed for surface cavity preparation (e.g. Komet, GEBR. BRASSELER sets 4337 and 4383):

- a small, non-adjustable head,

- different grain sizes for reduction control

- a long, slender neck for a direct view of the preparation,

- a slim profile for good irrigation in narrow cavities

- a rigid hold in the rotary head [66] (Figure 45).

However, to avoid neck breakage, it is preferable to use them with a red ring contra-angle at a maximum speed of 160,000 rpm, at low pressure and accompanied by a spray[66] .

- ◆ **Set 4337 contains :**
  - Smaller burs (889M/ 838M/ 830RM) are used to treat groove caries, or to access larger lesions.
  - Bulb-shaped burs (953M/ 953AM) are used for curettage of deeper caries.
  - The 830M/ 953M/ 953AM milling cutters can also access proximal faces more easily[66] .
- ◆ **Set 4383** is specially designed for excavating infected dentine. It contains two types of burr:
  - Tungsten carbide burs offer greater cutting efficiency, less heat generation and a smoother surface.
  - Diamond burs for sculpting and polishing fillings[66] .

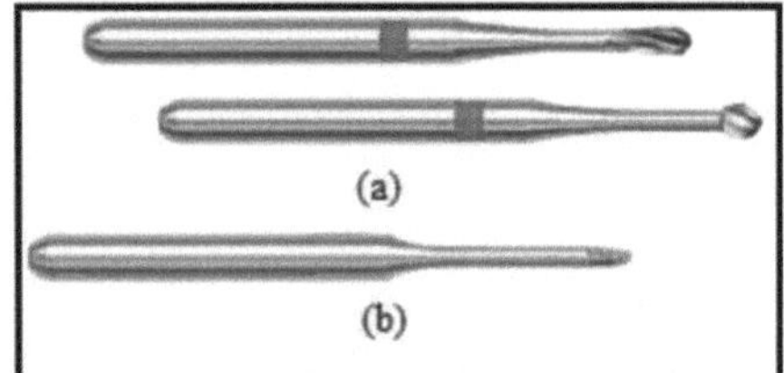

Figure 45: Micro burs: (a) Tungsten carbide burs, (b) Diamond burs [66]

Clinical application of micro burs (Figure 46):

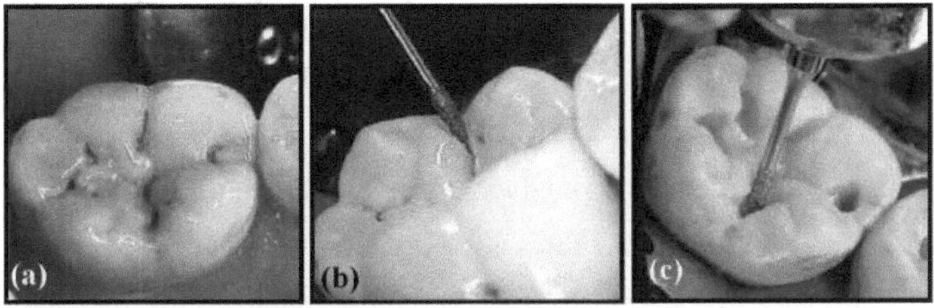

Figure 46: Use of microbeams on a 46: (a) Sillion caries and proximal caries;(b) Opening and exposure of the caries with the tip of the 889M instrument;(c) Excavation of the caries from the sulcus with the pear-shaped 830RM.314.009 instrument. [66]

6.2. Cutters made of self-limiting polymers

These burs have been developed to solve the clinical problem of the excavation limit point, the principle of which is based on the hardness of tooth structure rather than its coloring. They are made from self-limiting polymers whose specific Knoop hardness enables them to selectively remove carious dentine without affecting the integrity of the harder, healthy dentine. Example: SmartBurs II from SS White[23] (Figure 47).

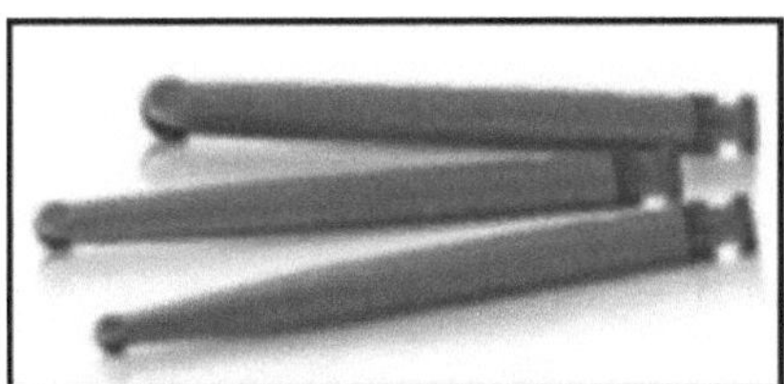

Figure 47: SmartBurs II milling cutters from the SS White laboratory []23

6. The air-abrasion technique

This technique involves the projection of abrasive particles by a high-velocity jet of compressed air to kinetically prepare the cavities. It was developed in 1945 by Robert Black as a replacement for the handpiece. It was subsequently diverted from its primary use in favor of diagnostic techniques, since at the time, the requirements of amalgam placement necessitated architectural preparations [7].

Nowadays, thanks to the concept of minimally invasive dentistry and adhesive filling materials, the use of this technique is becoming very attractive, offering several clinical advantages.

Air abrasion respects the principles of tissue economy, preserving the integrity of healthy tooth structures around the lesion.

It is a minimally invasive technique that allows small cavity preparations with rough surfaces ideal for direct bonding filling materials [50]. In addition, the lack of noise, vibration and heat generation causes less pain and reduces the need for and use of anaesthetics, making it well accepted by patients [7].

6.3. Mechanism of action

The air abrasion technique is based on the physical principles of kinetic energy and the dispersion effect of particles according to the formula $E= \frac{1}{2} mv^2$ (where "m" represents mass and "v" represents velocity) [22].

Control of the system by the operator is essential, as he has to deal with several variables in order to optimize the cutting efficiency of these abrasives. These include :

◆ **Particle shape :**

- angular ground powder,
- spherical [7]

Angular particles are more abrasive on hard tissue. However, in soft tissue, they are absorbed and lose their kinetic energy, unlike spherical particles, which do not penetrate and preserve their kinetic energy for destructuring and destroying the tissue [3].

◆ **Particle size :**

This only applies to spherical particles up to 150 microns in diameter [7]. Increasing particle size increases the kinetic energy transferred to the surface, which may cause discomfort for the patient. For this reason, a particle size of 27 μm has been deemed sufficient for intraoral preparations [3].

◆ **The nature of particles :**

Either alumina oxide(Ah03): These are biocompatible, hydrophobic particles with diameters between 27 and 50 μm.

They provide a hardness of 2100 knoop, necessary for abrasion at relatively low cost [3].

Or bioactive glasses: in powder or spherical form, with a hardness of 420 knoop less than that of alumina.

These bioactive glasses are fragile. Once in contact with hard tissue, they fracture and react with an aqueous or chemical solution. This leads to a structural change resulting in the formation of a surface layer of hydroxyapatite (HCA), hence the potential for remineralization of the surface [3].

Or polycarboxylate resin: This is a crushed powder whose hardness is slightly less than that of alumina but identical to that of dentin, allowing it to target soft tissue while sparing healthy tissue[3] .

◆ **Delivered pressure :**

Air pressure can reach 160 PSI (pounds per square inch). Knowing that lower pressures allow better control and visibility, Imran et al. suggest an air pressure of between 40 and 60 PSI (2.75-11.03 bar)[22] .

◆ **Insert diameter :**

Generally, there are two diameters to choose from: 0.38 or 0.48 mm.

According to Peruchi et al, the 0.48 mm tip increases the depth of preparation. Whereas the 0.38 mm tip enables precise tissue removal from temporary teeth[70] .

◆ **Insert angulation :**

■ 80° angulation:

As the jet is perpendicular to the surface, it concentrates the particles for maximum efficiency.

The cavity created in the enamel will be 39 to 169 um deep.

- ■ 45° angulation :

The oblique spray does not allow particles to be concentrated in one spot, as they will not hit the surface at the same time.

The cavity created will be shallower but wider[74] .

- ◆ **The distance between the nozzle and the surface to be treated :**

The operating distance should be between 0.5 and 2 mm to maximize the convergence of the abrasive jet. Beyond this value, the particles will disperse and lose cutting efficiency[22] .

- ◆ **Exposure time :**

The depth of preparation is proportional to the exposure time. For this reason, the practitioner is obliged to work in small strokes of 0.5-2 seconds and to make frequent checks to avoid over-preparation[3] .

- ◆ **Type of abrasive jet :**
  - ■ **Dry:** Dry abrasive air is very powerful but creates a lot of dust, which can abrade peripheral instrumentation[51] .
  - ■ **Wet:** The addition of water to our system concentrates the flow of particles and produces a precise abrasive jet that generates neither heat nor dust. This facilitates particle suction while preserving the vacuum motor[51] .

Today, air abrasion adds value in all areas of conservative dentistry. It is the technique of choice for the preparation of small cavities in Class V as well as Class I (Figure 48), Class II by creating tunnel-type cavities, and Class III and IV where access is easy and anesthesia is not required[50] . In addition, the use of an aeropolisher with a sodium bicarbonate ($NaHCO_3$) suspension enables wells and fissures, as well as caries cavities, to be cleaned, thus facilitating visual examination[7] .

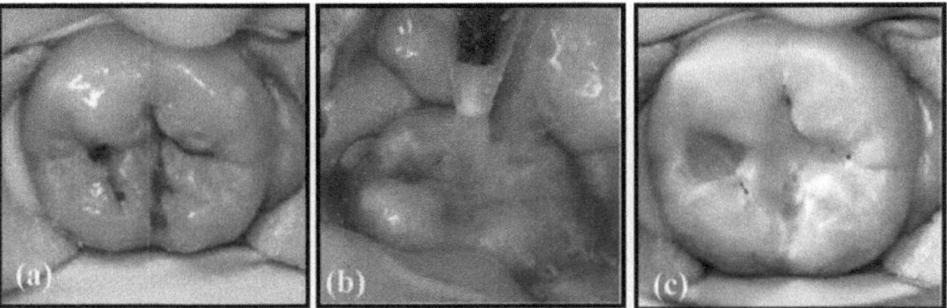

Figure 48: Preparing a cavity with moist air abrasion: (a) Class I carious lesion. (b) Cavity preparation. (c) Final result of preparation. [50]

7.2. The different systems

In the market, these systems can take the form of :

- a rolling accessory unit, such as the KCP-1000 whisper jet.
- a small scaler-type unit (e.g. Air flow® prep K1 MAX from EMS or L'AquaCare® from Velopex)
- a handpiece, such as Kavo's Rondoflex® plus (Figure 59) [51]

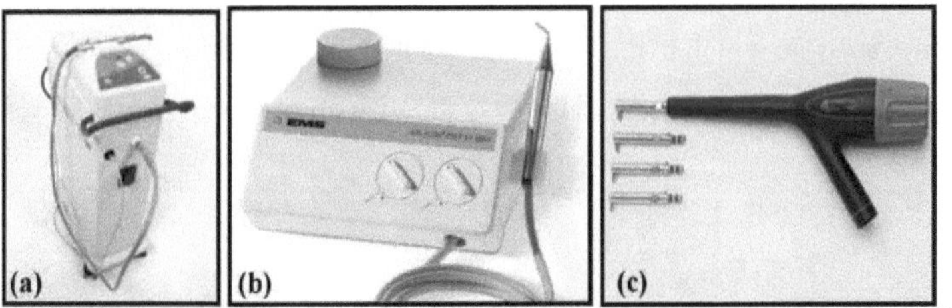

Figure 49: Different air abrasion systems: (a)KCP-1000 whisper jet. (b) Air flow® prep K1 MAX.(c) Rondoflex® plus [51]

However, there is a single-use dry air abrasion device that can be connected to the turbine cord via a special connection: Edge Dental's Airbrator® (Figure 50)[31] . The manufacturer provides a Starter Kit containing :

- the adapter for the turbine cord,
- color-coded abrasive cartridges:
  - ✓ **Red:** 3 high-grade alumina oxide cartridges
  - ✓ **Blue:** 1 medium-grain alumina oxide cartridge

✓ **Green:** 2 small-sized cartridges of sodium bicarbonate for polishing and cleaning [98]

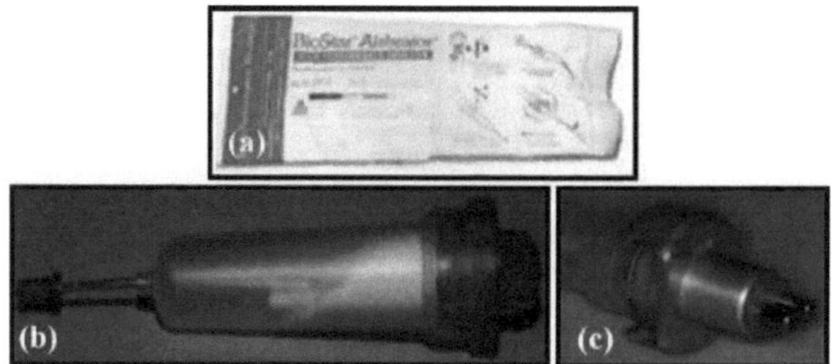

Figure 50: The Edge Dental Airbrator® (a) Storage bag with insertion instructions. (b) Disposable insert with high-grit cartridge;(c) Turbine cord adapter.[98]

7.3. Accessories for air abrasion devices

7.3.1. Air abrasion-resistant intraoral mirror

It has been designed by CrystalMark Dental Systems to withstand the indirect explosions of abrasive powder. This avoids the need for the dentist to check by direct vision, which in the long term would have deleterious effects on the back. The mirror is gold-plated for easy identification by staff[31] (Figure 51).

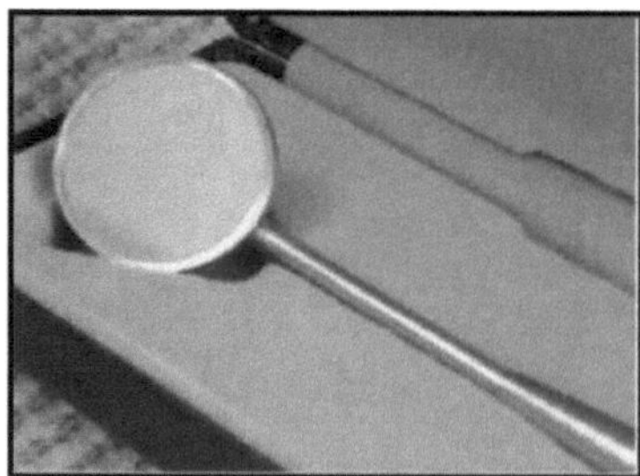

Figure 51: CrystalMark mirror [31]

7.3.2. Sand trap

This device enables abrasive particles to be evacuated through suction, preventing them from entering the patient's oral cavity (Figure52)[31] .

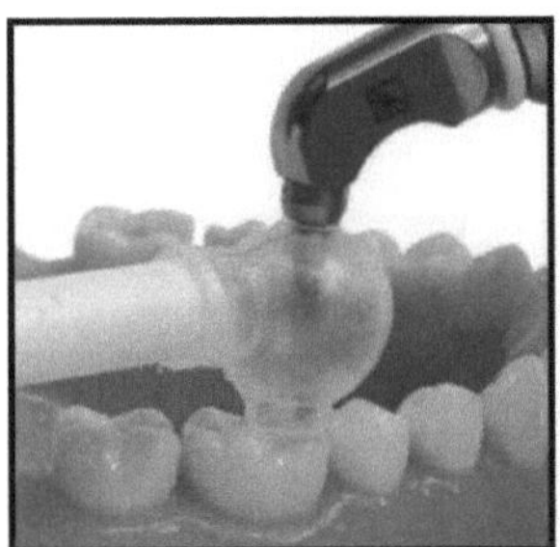

Figure 52: Particle trap [31]

7.3.3. Power plus booster

This accessory is available for Danville Engineering's Prep Start. It recompresses compressed air up to 135 ps, enabling faster cutting while reducing working time[31] .

7.3.4. High-volume exhaust system

This accessory is the ideal companion for abrasive air systems. It provides suction that eliminates any chance of contamination of the operation by abrasive particles. Example: the RapidVac[31] .

7.3.5. MicroVibe

It is a device whose tip provides mechanical vibrations that will facilitate the penetration of resin into narrow spaces and improve the sealing of pits and fissures by increasing the contact between the sealant and the tooth structure[31] .

8. Oscillatory systems

The technique uses two systems, sono abrasion and ultra sono abrasion, the principle of which is summed up in the use of an insert-type abrasive diamond instrument, animated by a vibratory movement on the carious lesion. This oscillating movement enables us to create complex "tunnel" or "funnel" cavities, finishes and other varied forms of preparation. What's more, the so-called hemiworking insert used has a working and a non-working side, which offers the advantage of preserving adjacent teeth during preparation of proximal cavities[83] (Figure 53).

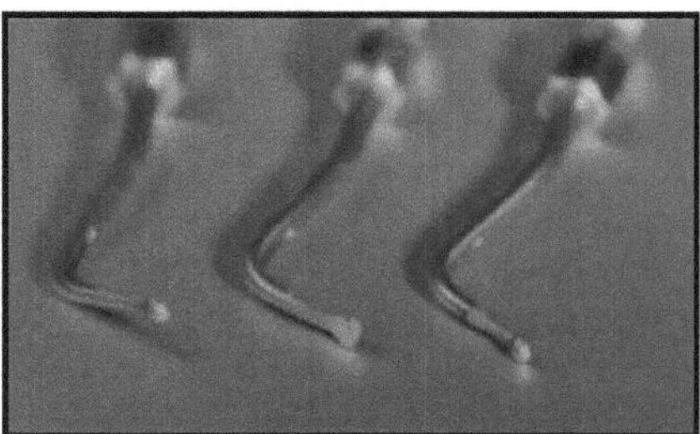

Figure 53: SONICflex inserts diamond-coated on one side only to allow minimal preparations [49]

8.1. Mechanism of action

The ultrasonic and sonic processes are orchestrated by four effects:

- **Vibration:** This generates the amplitude and path described by the insert. It is characterized by a frequency that regulates the instrument's impact on the tissue. It varies according to the power given by the generator, the insert used and the quantity of fluid used in combination: as fluid flow increases, vibration decreases.

- **Abrasion: This is** the mechanical effect associated with vibration. It depends on the grain size of the insert and the hardness of the tissue, following the gradient: enamel > altered enamel > dentin > cementum > decayed tissue > soft tissue.

So the harder the fabric, the more effective the abrasion.

- **Thermal effect: This** effect is a consequence of vibration and time of use. It is therefore recommended to use at least one irrigation alternately, and to work with intermittent contact to avoid heating the tissues.

- **Cavitation:** This corresponds to the implosion of microbubbles, formed by the waves, in the irrigation fluid. It plays an important role in cleaning surfaces and removing debris[16] .

8.1.1. Abrasive sound techniques

This technique generates vibrations using compressed air from the dental unit, which is transmitted to the handle of the handpiece. The pressurized air activates a pneumatic rotor to produce a circular oscillation, which is transmitted to the insert, which then works in a three-dimensional elliptical motion. The handpieces used operate at frequencies of 6000Hz with an amplitude of less than 200μm, delivering 3 power levels with a noise level of between 61 and 71dB (Table XII)[16] . Nowadays, they are equipped with integrated LEDs, a cooling spray and a multiplex connection[16] .

Table XII: SONICflex handpiece data sheet [83]

Power levels	Amplitude	Frequency	Noise level	Indications
Level 1	120 μm	6,000 Hz	61 dB	Finishing and tooth substance preservation
Level 2	160 μm	6,000 Hz	69 dB	Preparation
Level 3	160 μm	6,000 Hz	71 dB	Preparation with Approx inserts

8.1.2. Ultra sonic abrasive techniques

Note the existence of magnetostrictive ultrasound, which generates a vibration through an electric current transformed by magnetized blades. This is magnetostriction or "piezomagnetism", except that its application was oriented towards periodontal maintenance treatments, then gradually abandoned in favor of "piezoelectricity"[44] . The latter uses ultrasound of piezoelectric origin, which generates vibration through an alternating current amplified by a generator, conducted through ceramic pellets and transmitted to Tinsert, giving it a working capacity[16] . These ultrasonic handpieces deliver a high frequency of between 20,000Hz and 40,000Hz. They are equipped with LEDs and are used on piezoelectric generators with adjustable cooling spray and Tinsert vibration power to suit the application. Example: PIEZON® Master 700 from EMS (Figure 54)[16].

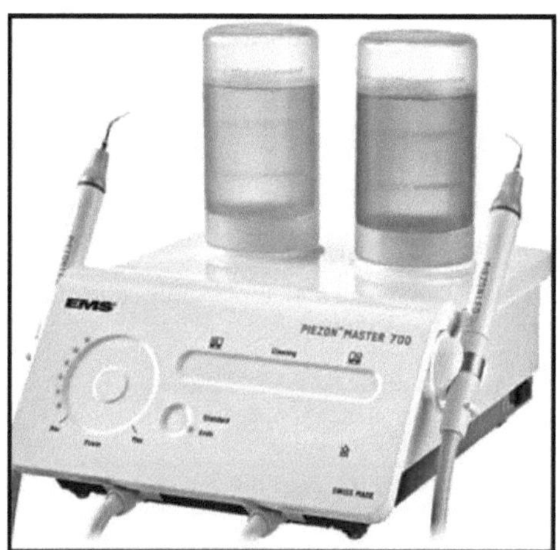

Figure 54: PIEZON® Master 700 from EMS [192]

8.2. Operating protocols

Preparation is limited to localized enamel access, followed by removal of underlying pathological dentine confined to the outer third of the dentin. In the most favourable cases, these two operations can be carried out concomitantly, by selecting a single sono-abrasive insert of suitable size and dimension. In general, this eviction is not completed by milling. Nevertheless, Tinsert's abrasion work can be facilitated by punctual ameliorative access, performed with a micro-dentistry diamond ball bur [16].

8.2.1. Mini occlusal cavities (wells, occlusal grooves)

As a general rule, for an anfractuous preparation strictly limited to the sulcus, a pointed insert with a working end should be chosen. On the other hand, if the lesion is localized in a fossa and extends in depth. Beyond the amelo-dentinal junction, we would choose a small-diameter ball or champagne cork insert [16] (Figure 55).

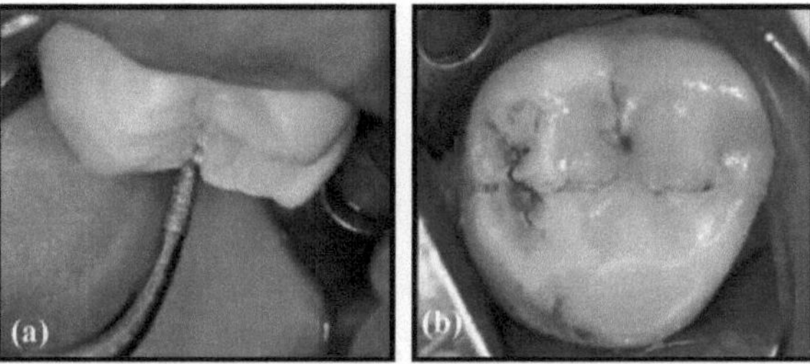

Figure 55: Preparation of a decayed distal occlusal groove of a 27: (a) Insert SF 849 009 SonicLineKometS in place; (b) Clinical result [16]

However, if the occlusal-distal grooves of maxillary molars are to be opened, there is a risk of over-preparation, compounded by the difficulty of access and vision. For this reason, it would be preferable to complete tissue removal by milling, using suitably sized ceramic burs (e.g. K1SM 204, CeraburKomet®) (010-012) (Figure 56).

The latter present a lower risk than conventional rotary instruments and limit the embrittlement of marginal ridges[16] .

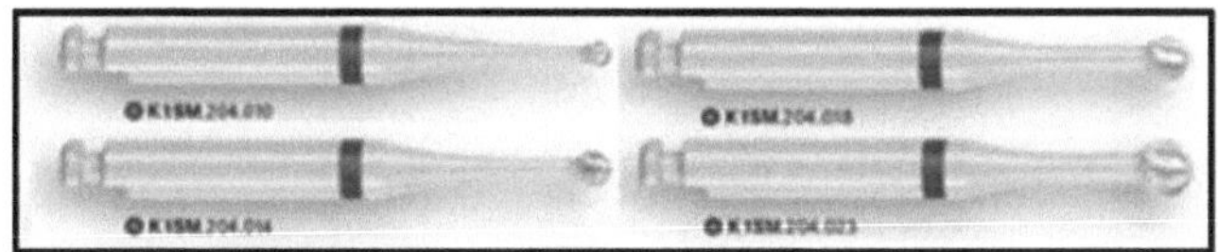

Figure 56: CeraburKomet® K1SM 204 ceramic burs [16]

In special cases, such as occlusal micro-preparation in the presence of carious erosive cavitations of the cusp tips, multi-blade ball inserts can be used to remove damaged tissue and prepare the enamel, while preventing micro-cracking and limiting embrittlement in areas subject to high mechanical stress[16] (Figure 57).

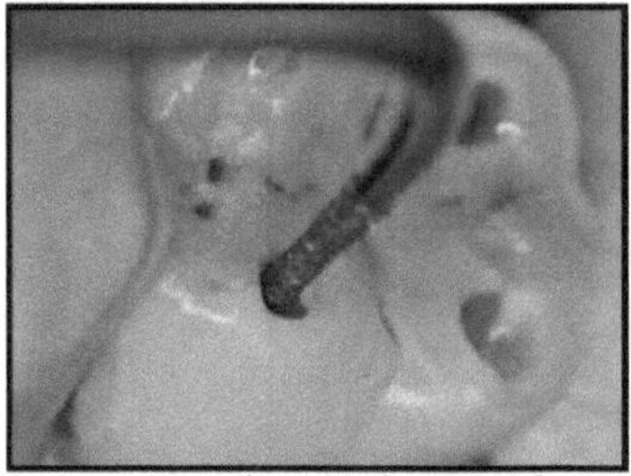

Figure 57: Occlusal micro-preparation with the 42 311 SonicflexKavoS insert [16]

8.2.2. Proximal mini-cavities

These preparations differ in that the marginal ridge is retained or partially removed.

◆ Preparation with partial removal of the marginal ridge

The standard procedure consists of :

- Use a diamond bur to gain access to the enamel.

- Select the type of insert and the mesial or distal orientation of its diamond-tipped working part to complete the preparation.

- Simultaneously create the "mini-cavity" and finish the cervical and proximal edges[16] (figure 58).

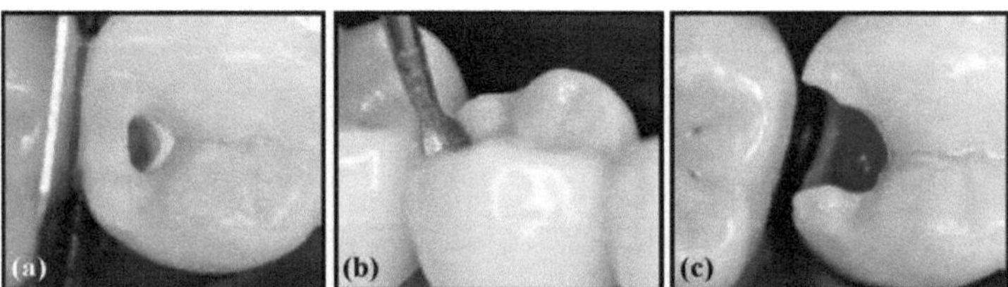

Figure 58: Performing a proximal micro-preparation with the 33 SonicSys micro Kavo® hemispherical insert. (a) Enamel access with diamond bur; (b) Removal of altered tissue; (d) Final result of preparation.[16]

It is worth noting that despite the use of hemiworking inserts, which offer us the advantage of preserving adjacent teeth, it would be wise to install a matrix and wedge protection: example Fender Wedge Prep Directa ®[16] .

◆ **Preparation with partial preservation of the marginal ridge :**

Two types of preparation are available:

- An occluso-proximal tuned slot preparation: **This** is a vertical proximal mini-cavity, which is considered to be the interproximal adhesive preparation of first intention, in the concept of *a minima* operative treatment of SiSta 2.1 and 2.2 carious lesions [1 6].

- Preparation via vestibulo-lingual access: a horizontal mini-cavity.

These types of preparation are reserved for the following special cases:

- Or a lesion distant from the interproximal contact.

- Or direct access to the lesion, thanks to the absence of an adjacent tooth.

- A very triangular embrasure with a high Le Huche index.

- Or a malposition [1 6].

Nevertheless, whatever the type of access, the practitioner must operate under a dam to displace the interdental papilla, and with optical aids to guide the insert into areas of carious extension and control the progressive elimination of$_{durs}$ tissues [16].

8.2.3. Mini cervical cavities

These preparations are facilitated by direct access to the lesion in the cervical third of the vestibular and lingual surfaces, and can be performed using a half-ball sono-abrasive insert.

The latter can easily work in the embrasure if lesions extend proximally, allowing us to selectively subtract non-conservable enamel and/or dentin, while preserving periodontal tissues (Figure 59) [1 6]. For aesthetic reasons, we can :

- Chamfer the cavosuperficial edge of the overlying enamel

- Or peel off as little as possible of an altered, blackish dentinal surface [1 6].

According to the Meta analysis by Ntovas et al in 2017, beveling inaccessible cervical margins improves marginal adaptation [68].

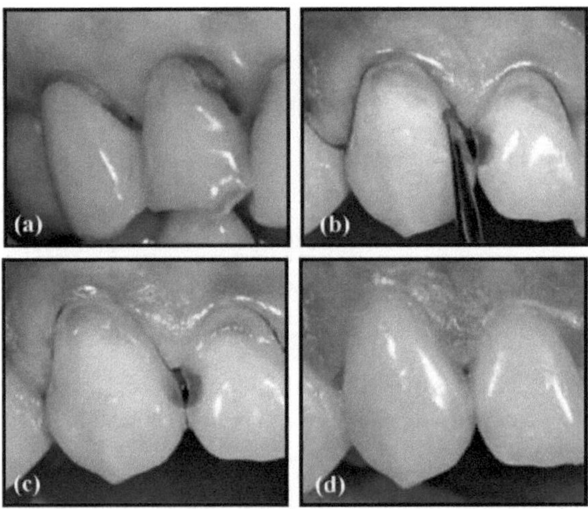

Figure 59: Sono-abrasive preparations of cervical lesions:(a) Secondary juxtagingival carious lesions of site 3.(b) Use of half-ball diamond insert.(c) Final result of preparations (d) Clinical result after composite restorations.[16]

Giuriato et al, in an in vitro study, compared the degree of microinfiltration of Class V composite resin restorations whose cavities were made on 30 bovine teeth divided into three treatment groups (n = 10): G1 - preparation with a diamond bur, G2 - preparation with Er, Cr: YSGG laser (2.78 µm) and G3 - preparation with diamond tips attached to the ultrasonic system (CVDentus) . The treatment results for the 3 groups showed a significant difference (p = 0.0007). However, the effectiveness of the ultrasonic system was not statistically significantly different from that of the diamond burr (p> 0.05)[27] .

9. The laser

9.1. Laser light presentation

9.1.1. Composition of laser light

It's a light that doesn't exist in nature, but results from the amplification of light by stimulated emission of radiation, which depends on the coexistence of three elements (Figure 60):

- **An active medium**: this is made up of the atoms you wish to excite, and is represented either by a gas (CO_2, neon helium, Argon), a solid (Nd- YAG, Er-YAG) or a liquid (dyes).

- This is the medium that will enable us to define the type of laser.

- **A pumping source**: this is an external source that supplies the medium with initial energy, enabling molecular excitation and thus the conversion of low-energy atoms into high-energy atoms: this is known as "population inversion".

- **A resonance cavity**: this is created by placing two flat or spherical mirrors face to face, spaced at a distance L depending on the wavelength produced. This makes it possible to reflect certain light rays that might otherwise remain confined [11].

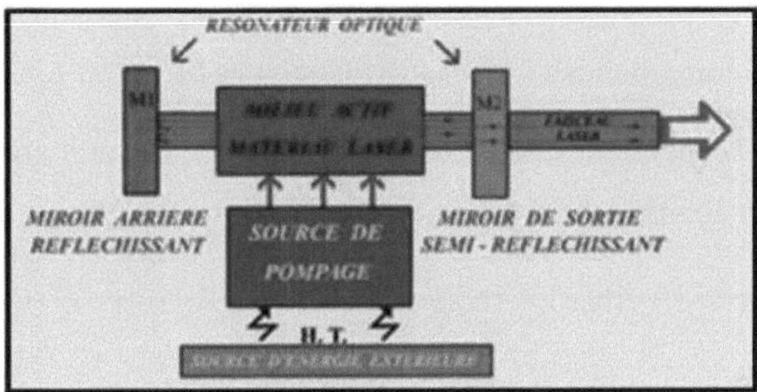

Figure 60: Laser operating principle [96]

9.1.2. Properties of laser light

The resulting laser beam is unidirectional, monochromatic, coherent and intense [1 1]. Most laser beams are emitted in the visible or infrared range (Figure 61) [26].

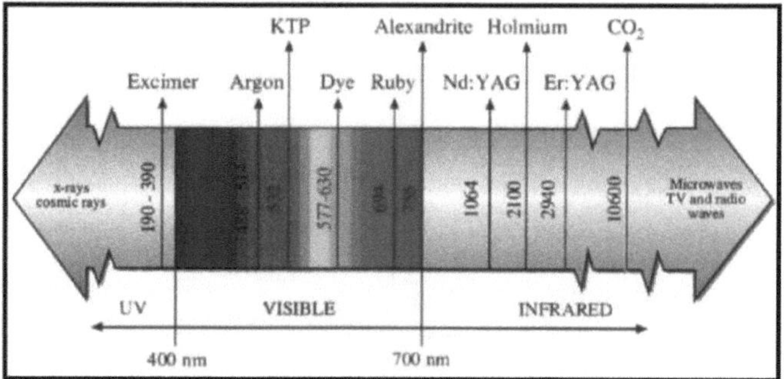

Figure 61: The spectrum of different lasers [26]

9.1.3.　　　Energy characteristics of laser light

The energies generated are measured according to :

- **Power**: measured in watts (W). It represents the power of an energy system in which an energy of 1 joule is uniformly transferred for 1 second ($W=J.s^{\wedge}$).[1]

- **Energy:** expressed in Joules (J), this characterizes the work produced by a system to generate light, heat or motion.

I   joule corresponds to exposure to a power of 1 watt for one second.

- **Fluence**: the amount of energy received per unit area, expressed in J/cm^2 [75] .

II   There are 3 emission modes:

- **Continuous:** instantaneous power is constant over time.

- **Pulse or pulsed:** instantaneous power varies with time.

■ **Triggered:** interruption of continuous beam[75] .

9.2. Areas of use

It should be noted that, depending on wavelength and tissue composition, the laser beam may react in different ways: it will be transmitted, reflected, absorbed or scattered (Figure 62)[80] .

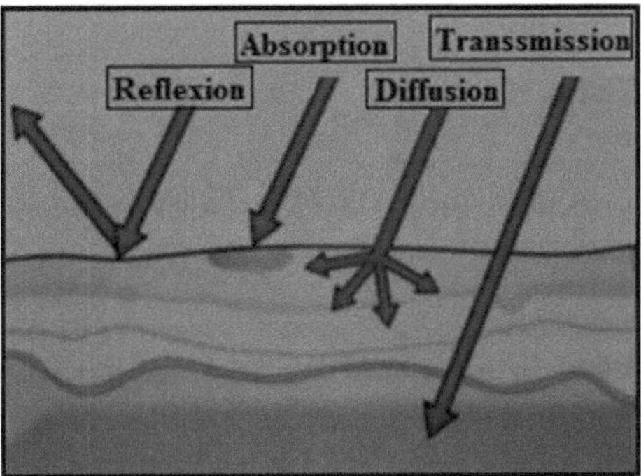

Figure 62: Interactions between laser beams and tissue [80]

However, when directed at dental, gingival or bone tissue, several effects are obtained, distinguished as follows (Figure 63):

The effects of laser radiation absorbed at the surface of tissues :

■ **Photo-ablation**: this involves the breaking of molecular bonds.

■ Or **heating**: this is a thermal effect resulting in liquefaction and vaporization of tissues following an increase in temperature due to molecular vibrations.

The effects of laser radiation penetrating deep into tissues :

■ Or **decontamination**: this eliminates the pathogenic bacteria responsible for a wide range of infections.

■ **Cellular bio-stimulation:** desensitizing, anti-inflammatory and analgesic effect.

■ Or **bio-activation:** activation and acceleration of bone or gingival healing[26] .

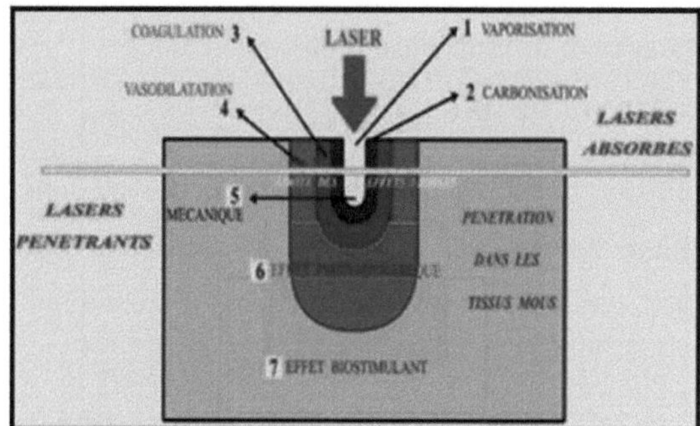

Figure 63: The main effects of lasers [96]

We note that each wavelength has a specific absorption in the various constituents of biological tissues: water, hemoglobin, hydroxyapatite and melanin [80] (Figure 64).

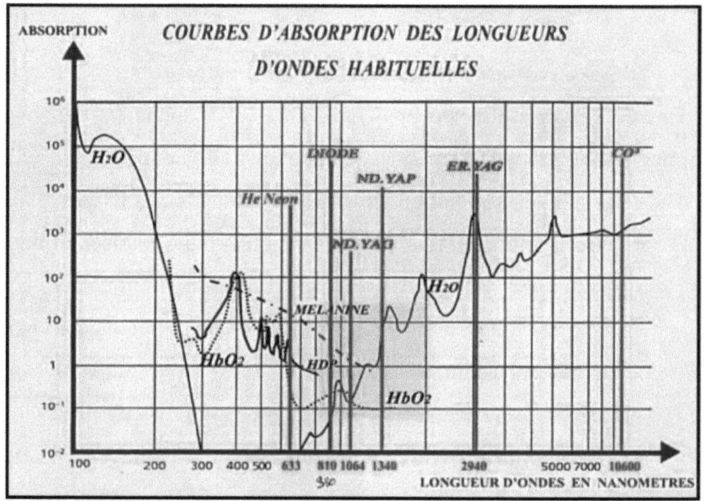

Figure 64: Absorption diagram for lasers in the various constituents of biological tissue [80].

Consequently, the specific characteristics and wavelengths of each laser will be decisive in influencing their affinity for the different tissues in the oral cavity (Table XIII) [80].

The different lasers	Wavelength (λ)	Affinity	Indications
The KTP laser	$\lambda =$ 532nm	o Pigments o Hemoglobin	o Coagulation o Clarification
The diode laser	$\lambda =$ 650nm	o Water o Hemoglobin	o Periodontology o Soft tissue surgery o Coagulation, o Lighting
Nd: YAG Nd: YAP	$\lambda=1064$nm $\lambda=1340$nm	o Pigments	Soft tissue surgery
Er, Cr-YSGG	$\lambda =$ 2780nm	o Water o Hydroxyapatite	Soft and hard tissue surgery
Er: YAG	$\lambda = 2940$ nm	o Water o Hydroxyapatite	Soft and hard tissue surgery
CO2 laser	$\lambda=10600$ nm	o Water	Soft tissue surgery

In conservative dentistry, the phenomenon exploited in minimally invasive procedures is none other than the photo-ablation of hard tissue, achieved by transferring high energy to the water it contains.

This phenomenon produces a slight noise due to the explosion of water molecules, earning it the name "explosive vaporization" [80].

According to Bertrand and Rocca, the action of an Erbium YAG laser on enamel and dentin results from the absorption of radiation in water and apatite crystals (Figure 65). Bearing in mind that pathological tissues are the most water-saturated, and that enamel is the most mineralized tissue in the body (around 97% hydroxyapatite crystals), more so than dentin (70%), which on the other hand is much richer in water, they concluded that it is the laser of choice for the preparation of hard tissues (enamel, dentin, bone, cementum) and for the removal of carious tissue [10].

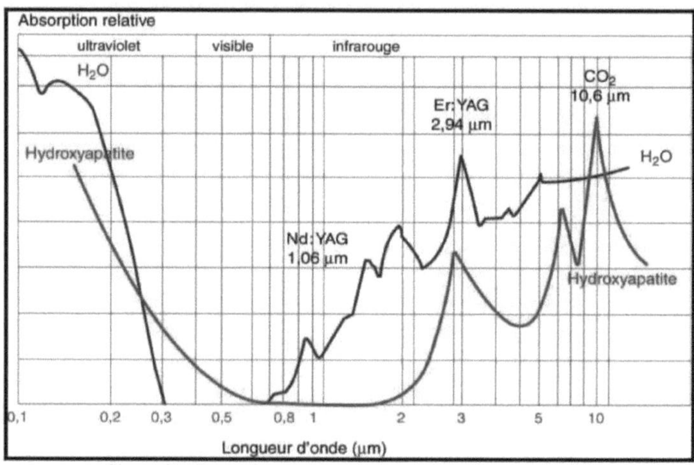

Figure 65: Absorption spectra of water and hydroxyapatite [10]

9.3. The Er:YAG laser

9.3.1. Presentation

The Er:YAG laser emits in the mid-infrared at a wavelength of 2,940 nm. The active medium is a Y3Al5O12 aluminum yttrium garnet doped with Erbium ions^{+3} . Pumping is achieved with a very intense flash of light corresponding to an absorption band of the Er^{+3} ion incorporated in the[10] crystal. In omni-practice, the Er-YAG laser is considered the most versatile (Figure 66).

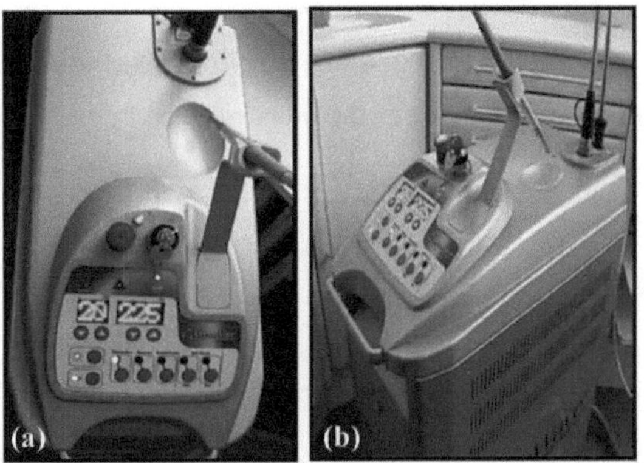

Figure 66: Er-YAG laser on carriage: (a) Front view; (b) Side view. [80]

Transmission takes place in very short pulses of the order of 240 microseconds, interspersed with rest periods, and the energy of each pulse can be adjusted by the operator[80] . As for transmission, this can be achieved either via a flexible optical fiber, which is easy to handle but fragile, or via an articulated arm, which is slightly bulkier but more robust. The latter has a minimal energy loss, unlike the fiber, which has a relatively high energy loss of around 60%(Figure 67)[10] .

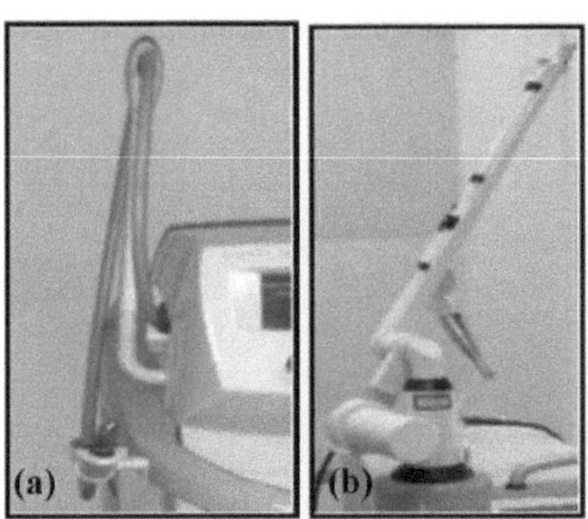

Figure 67: Types of laser beam transmission: (a). Flexible optical fiber (Key 3™,Kavo). (b) Articulated arm (Fidelis Plus™, Fotona) i[10

At the end, an optical contra-angle will be mounted, which will ensure transmission in different ways:

- ■ **Either non-contact**: transmission is ensured by a mirror with a focal distance to be respected of the order of 9 to15 mm below or above which there is a risk of losing some of the ablation potential (Figure 68)[10]

.

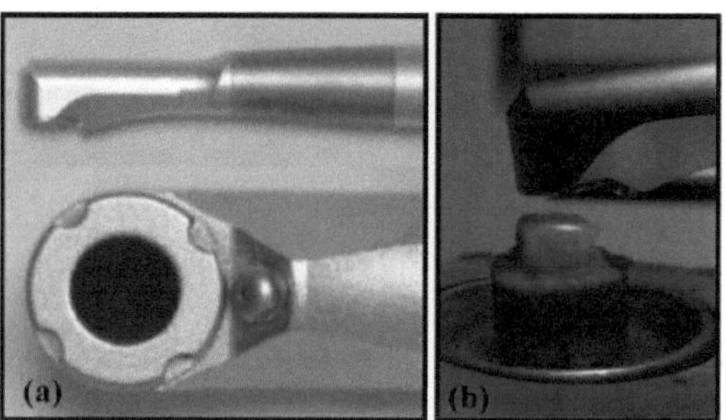

Figure 68: Non-contact laser transmission:(a)Optical contra-angle 2060™, Kavo (b)Remote mirror transmission[10].

- ■ **Either contact**: transmission is provided by a special quartz or sapphire **tip** (Figure 69)[10] .

It should be noted that for practical reasons, to facilitate the practitioner's work, a red guiding beam is used as infra-reds are not visible to the naked eye[80] .

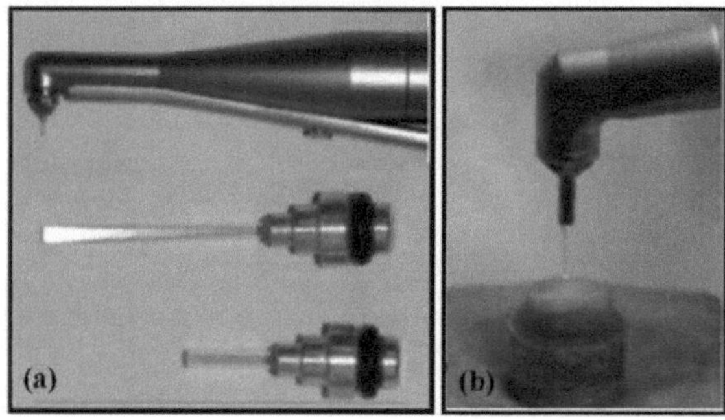

9.3.2. Clinical benefits

◆ **Visibility:**

As modern micro-dentistry is based on the principles of tissue economy, the dentist is obliged to continuously monitor his work (Figure 70).

Accompanying ourselves with a continuous spray of water allows us to cool and clean the work area, which preserves the underlying healthy tissue [42].

Studies by Dostalova et al. on surface modifications on enamel and dentin showed that Er:YAG laser irradiation without water spray caused microcracks on the enamel edges of the cavity, whereas laser irradiation with water spray did not, and ablation remained localized, with no identified thermal damage to enamel or surrounding dentin [19].

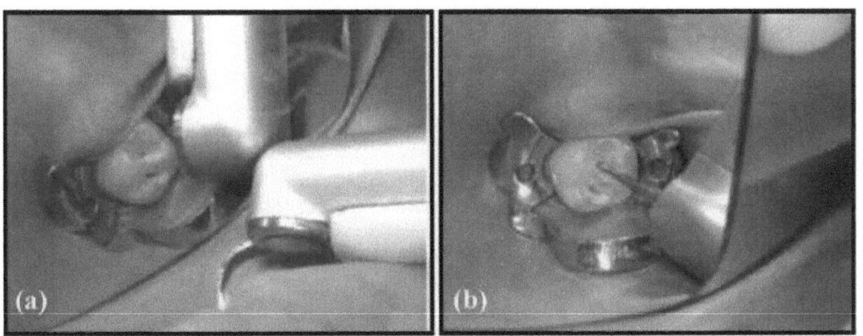

Figure 70: Comparison of the visibility of conventional and laser treatments: (a) Good visibility with the Er: YAG laser (b)Poor visibility with conventional curettage [42].

◆ **Preparation efficiency:**

The choice to use Er-YAG in conservative dentistry stems from its high absorption in water and in apatite crystals, while presenting a low tissue penetration power of between 2 and 15 microns. This explains its high efficacy on hard tissue (Figure 71) [80]. This effectiveness was studied and confirmed by Hadley et al., who compared the different preparations of class

I, III and V cavities performed with a conventional air turbine with those using the erbium, chromium: Er, Cr: YSGG laser [30].

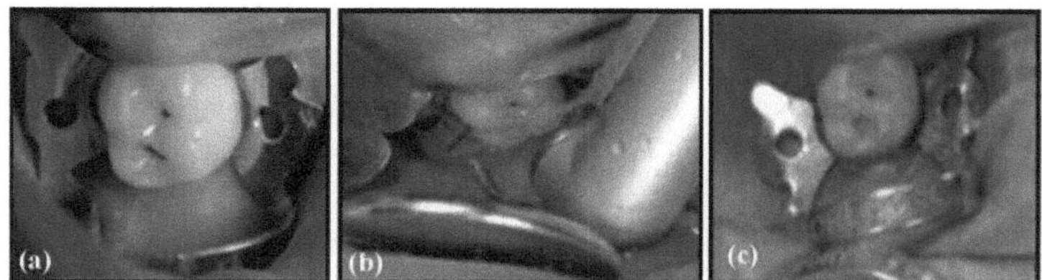

Figure 71: Laser treatment: (a) Placement of an operating field;(b) Laser curettage; (c) Result of the cavity. [42]

These lasers have been shown to be suitable for tunneling-type adhesive micro-dentistry techniques (Figure 72)[26] .

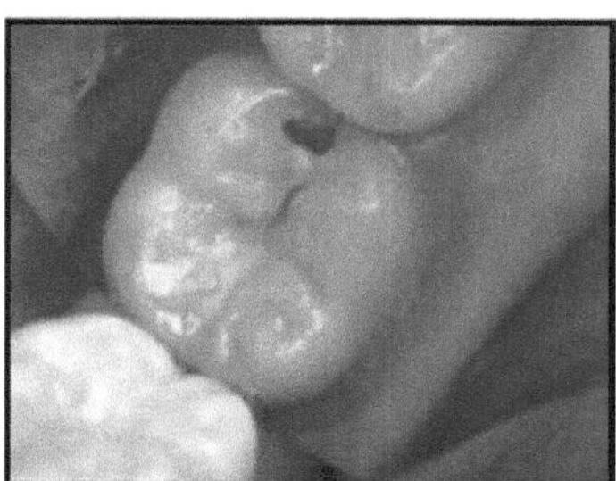

Figure 72: Creating a tunnel cavity with an Er-YAG laser [ ]26

The 2017 meta-analysis by Tao et Coll, aimed to compare the efficacy of erbium laser technology versus the traditional milling technique in the removal of carious tissue. They deduced that caries curettage time was increased with Erbium lasers compared to milling (mean difference: 3.48 min, with 95% confidence interval: [1.90-5.06], P <0.0001). However, erbium laser technology reduced the need for local anesthesia (hazard ratio: 0, 28, with 95% confidence interval: [0.13-0.62], P
= 0,002). This allows us to make up for lost time, as the session starts immediately[81] .

◆ **Patient comfort:**

The Er/YAG laser is particularly popular with patients who associate pain with auditory aggression, and is finding success with younger patients[89] .

In 2014, Zhegova and Rashkova conducted a clinical study on adolescents aged between 16 and 18 years, with the aim of assessing their acceptance and perception of pain during conventional mechanical preparations compared to those using an Er-YAG laser. They found that none of the children requested a local anaesthetic during preparation, and the results were such that 86.36% of them preferred laser preparation and wished to use it for future treatments[89] (Figure 73 and 74).

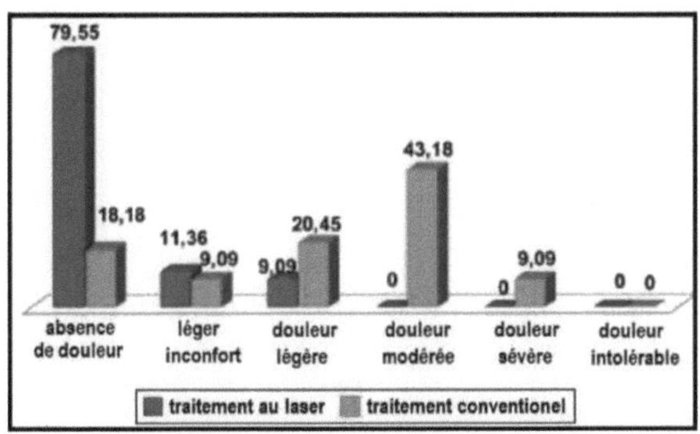

Figure 73: Percentage distributions of children according to their perceptions of pain during caries treatment [89].

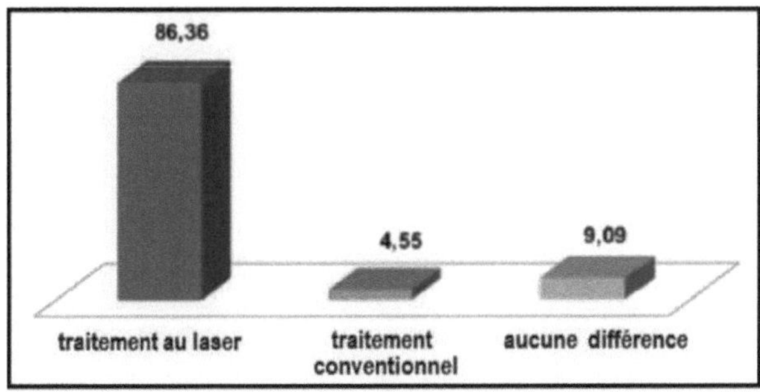

Figure 74: Representative diagram of future treatment methods for children according to their preferences[8 9]

According to Tao et Coll's 2017 meta-analysis, vibration, sight and sound, which were the most common nuisance factors in patients during conventional cavity preparation, were eliminated with lasers :

- Prevalence of vibrations in the milling/laser group: 86.7%, 2.2%.

- Prevalence of sight in milling/laser groups: 40%, 20%.

- Prevalence of sound in the milling/laser group: 62.2%, 15.6%.

However, the smell and taste during laser preparation increased:

- Prevalence of odour in milling/laser group: 17.8%, 66.7%.

- Prevalence of taste in milling/laser group: 22.2%, 42.2%.

As for postoperative pain, the study showed no significant difference between the two treatment groups (RR = 0.80, 95% CI: [0.17, 3.88], P = 0.78)[81] .

◆ Bactericidal effect :

The action of the Erbium laser enables us to obtain a clean cavity, free from dentin sludge and bacterial debris.

Indeed, various microbiological studies have been carried out by authors such as Folwaczny in 2007 or Schoop et al in 2004, to test the bactericidal effect of different lasers. They revealed the absence of bacteria up to 1 mm into dentin. Results obtained with the Er: YAG laser showed a complete reduction in E. Coli in 75% of samples, as well as a reduction in *E. Faecalis*. They concluded that this system is suitable for decontaminating the dentin surface during cavity preparation, compared with conventional methods where it is difficult to eliminate dentin infection even after all decayed tissue has been removed[42] . This disinfection of contaminated dentine reduces the risk of caries recurrence[26] .

Other authors, such as Baraba et Coll in 2018, have further evaluated the effectiveness of these Er- YAG lasers in eliminating cariogenic bacteria and carious dentin by varying their pulse modes, with a secondary objective of measuring temperature during caries tissue ablation through an infrared thermal camera.

The study was carried out using two lasers: a first Er: YAG laser controlled by fluorescence-feedback (FFC) and a second Er: YAG laser based on variable square pulse (VSPt) technology. Seventy-two extracted human molars were used randomly in 4 groups:

- group 1: 400 ms (FFC group);
- group 2: short super pulse (SSP group, 50 ms pulse);
- group 3: short medium pulse (MSP group, 100 ms pulse);
- group 4: short pulse (SP group, 300 ms pulse)

Post-treatment results from all groups were free from bacterial contamination. While temperatures measured in the SSP, MSP and SP groups were significantly higher compared to temperatures in the FFC group (P<0.001) without being excessive to adversely affect pulp health (Figure 75)[9] .

According to Bertrand and Rocca, the Er-YAG laser keeps the rise in intra-pulpal temperature well below the biologically acceptable threshold of 5°C[10] .

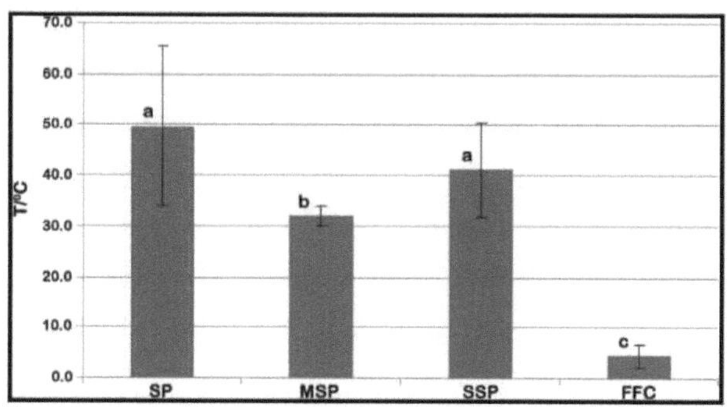

Figure 75: Mean temperature (C°) and standard deviations for the FFC, SP, MSP and SSP groups [9]

◆ Compatibility with adhesive systems :

When using the Er:YAG laser, microscopic observations showed the absence of dentin sludge and debris, as well as the presence of numerous microscopic reliefs associated with greater removal of inter-tubular dentin[10] . In the literature, it has been suggested that this prepared surface is sterile from the outset and will not require selective etching, and the adhesive system can be applied directly[10] . Nowadays, however, the irradiated enamel must be pre-treated with orthophosphoric acid before composite bonding.

Setien et al tested the watertightness of composite restorations on class V cavities prepared with an Er:YAG laser with or without acid application and using a silver nitrate solution.

The results showed that only the non-acid-treated samples showed a loss of enamel seal, without the dye exceeding the enamel thickness[10] .

Visuri et al. used an Er:YAG laser at 350 mJ/pulse and 6 Hz with an application of a 10% phosphoric acid solution for 30 seconds.

They obtained a higher shear strength for dentin treated only with the Er:YAG laser. They concluded that no acid pretreatment of dentin was necessary before bonding a composite resin[10] .

However, Ceballos et al. used the same protocol, but with an Er-YAG laser with an energy of 180 mJ/pulse and a frequency of 2 Hz, together with an application of 35% orthophosphoric acid for 15 seconds. They obtained higher values for dentin irradiated and then subjected to the action of the acid than for dentin subjected solely to the action of laser radiation[10] .

This latter study was confirmed by Bertrand and Rocca, who evaluated the watertightness of Class V cavity composite restorations prepared with the Er:YAG laser at a displayed energy of 500 mJ/pulse 10 Hz, under a spray of water (fluence: 44.2 J/cm2) while systematizing the use of acid. The results of composite restorations placed in cavities prepared with the Er:YAG laser and then treated with 35% ortho-phosphoric acid for 15 seconds were the least sensitive to dye infiltration (Figure 76)[10] .

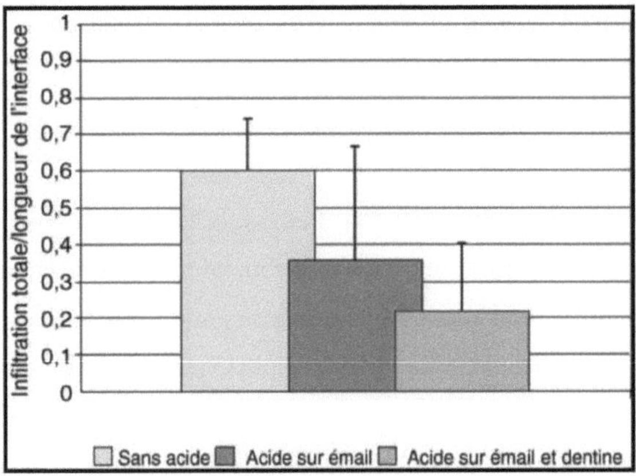

Figure 76: Sealing of Class V cavity composite resin restorations prepared with an Er:YAG laser [10].

According to tao et Co's 2017 meta-analysis, restorative loss shows no significant difference between milling systems and lasers: RR = 0.90, 95% CI: [0.21, 3.84], P = 0.89[81] .

Conclusion

In recent decades, the evolving concept of microdentistry has contributed to a change in approach to the management of carious lesions.

This evolution has been accompanied by the emergence of new classifications that take into account the stage of the carious lesion, such as the ICDAS and SISTA classifications. Technological advances have also played a key role in the development and improvement of diagnostic tools.

Today's dentists use not only traditional diagnostic tools, but also innovative devices such as transillumination, impedance, electrical conductivity and ultrasound, to make more precise diagnoses and offer more appropriate treatment.

In the case of early, non-cavitating carious lesions, reversionary treatments such as remineralization with fluoride, remineralization with amorphous calcium phosphate-casein phosphopeptide (CPP-ACP) and ozone therapy are recommended.

But if these prove impossible, new non-invasive treatments, such as resin micro-infiltration, may be indicated.

Furthermore, techniques such as chemo-mechanical curettage or anti-traumatic restorative treatment (ART) for incipient cavitary carious lesions are in line with the principles of micro-dentistry and rarely require anesthesia, which is a major advantage for children and anxious adult patients.

When it comes to working on dental tissue, the dentist's therapeutic arsenal includes ultra-conservative treatment methods such as micro-mills, specially designed for the preparation of superficial cavities, air-abrasion systems, oscillatory systems (sono or ultrasonic abrasion) and ER-YAG lasers.

However, the field of dentistry is constantly evolving, and the cost of these procedures is still too high for the general public. This raises the question of whether the democratization of these procedures will become obsolete as we move into the new era of regenerative dentistry and tissue engineering.

References

1. **Alammari MR, Smith PW, De Jong EDJ.** Quantitative light-induced fluorescence (QLF): a tool for early occlusal dental caries detection and supporting decision making in vivo. *JDent 2013;41(2):127-32.*

2. **Al-Swaidy MH, Salih BA.** Efficacy of papacarie in reduction total bacterial count in comparison with the conventional rotary method. *J Baghdad Coll Dent 2016;28(4):141-3.*

3. **Arvind A, Siddharth P, Kulwinder K.** A new dimension to conservative dentistry: air abrasion. *Indian JDent Sci 2014;6(22):124-7.*

4. **Azizi Z.** Management of white spot lesions using resin infiltration technique: a review. *Open JDent OralMed 2015;3(1):1-6.*

5. **Azrak B, Callaway A, Grundheber A,** Stender E, Willershausen B. Comparison of the efficacy of chemomechanical caries removal (Carisolv®) with that of conventional excavation in reducing the cariogenic flora. *Int J Paediatr Dent 2004;14(3): 182-91.*

6. **Bader JD, James D, Shugars DA.** A systematic review of the performance of a laser fluorescence device for detecting caries. *JAm Dent Assoc 2004;135(10):1413-26.*

7. **Banerjee A, Watson TF.** Air abrasion: its uses and abuses. *Dent Update 2002;29(7):340-6.*

8. **Banting D, Eggertsson H, EkstrandKR et al.** Rationale and evidence for the international caries detection and assessment system (ICDAS II). *Ann Arbor 2005;1001:48109-78.*

9. **Baraba A, Kqiku L, Gabric D, Verzak Z, Hanscho K, Miletic I.** Efficacy of removal of cariogenic bacteria and carious dentin by ablation using different modes of Er: YAG lasers. *Braz JMedBiol Res 2018;51(3):e6872*

10. **Bertrand MF, Rocca JP.** ER : YAG laser and restorative dentistry. *EMC- Stomatologie 2005;1(2):104-15.*

11. **Bertrand MF, Rocca JP.** Lasers in oral medicine. *Real Clin 2012;23:85-94*

12. **Chala S, Bouamara R, Abdallaoui F, Antoun Z.** Methods for diagnosing initial carious lesions. *Rev Odontstomatol 2004;33(4):297-310.*

13. **Clark MB, Slayton RL.** Fluoride use in caries prevention in the primary care setting. *JPediatr 2014;134(3):626-33.*

14. **Damen JJ, Buijs MJ, Ten Cate JM.** Acidogenicity of buccal plaque after a single rinse with amine fluoride-stannous fluoride mouthrinse solution. *Caries Res 2002;36(1):53-7.*

15. **De Oliveira AF, De Oliveira DL, Forte FD, Sampaio FC, Ccahuana- Vásquez RA, Amaechi BT.** In situ effect of a CPP-ACP chewing gum on enamel erosion associated or not with abrasion. *Clin Oral Investig 2017;21(1):339-46*

16. **Decup F, Lasfargues JJ.** Minimal adhesive preparations and restorations. Contribution of sono-abrasive techniques. *Real Clin 2012;23(3):1-12.*

17. **Denis M, Atlan A, Attal JP.** Erosion/infiltration: a new treatment for white spots. *Odontologie 2012;1:1-6.*

18. **Diniz MB, Rodrigues JA, Lussi A.** Traditional and novel caries detection methods. *Contemp Approach Dent Caries 2012;6:105-28.*

19. **Dostalova T, Jelinkova H, Kresja O, Hamal H.** Evaluation of the surface changes in enamel and dentin due to possibility of thermal overheating induced by erbium : YAG laser radiation. *Scanning Microsc 1996;10(1):285-91.*

20. **Eggertsson H, Analoui M, Van Der Veen MH, González-Cabezas C, Eckert GJ, Stookey GK.** Detection of early interproximal caries in vitro using laser fluorescence, dye-enhanced laser fluorescence and direct visual examination. *Caries Res 1999;33(3):227-33.*

21. **Ekstrand KR, Bakhshandeh A, Martignon S.** Treatment of proximal superficial caries lesions on primary molar teeth with resin infiltration and fluoride varnish versus fluoride varnish only: efficacy after 1 year. *Caries Res 2010;44(1):41-6.*

22. **Farooq I, Imran Z, Farooq U.** Air Abrasion: Truly Minimally Invasive Technique. *Int J Prosthodont Rest Dent 2011;1(2):105-7.*

23. **Freedman G.** Conservative dentistry in constant evolution. *Dent Trib Study Club 2013;1:36-40.*

24. **Frencken JE.** Atraumatic restorative treatment and minimal intervention dentistry. *Br Dent J 2017;223(3): 183-9.*

25. **Garcia-Godoy F, Hicks MJ.** Maintaining the integrity of the enamel surface: the role of dental biofilm, saliva and preventive agents in enamel demineralization and remineralization. *JAm Dent Assoc 2008;139:25-34.*

26. **Gaultier F, Navarro G.** Lasers in dentistry. *Le fil dentaire 2006;12:26- 30.*

27. **GiuriatoJB, Freitas PM, Nagaze DY, Oda M.** In vitro evaluation of microleakage in class V restorations after cavity preparation with high speed, ultrasonic and laser. *Clin Lab Res Dent 2014;20(1):39-45.*

28. **Guéders A, Geerts S.** Ozone: an alternative to surgical treatment of caries? *Act Dent Ulg 2007;37:23-33.*

29. **Guimerà A, Calderón E, Los P, Christie AM.** Method and device for bioimpedance measurement with hard-tissue applications. *Physiol Meas 2008;29(6):279-90.*

30. **Hadley J, Young DA, Eversole LR, Gombein JA.** A laser-powered hydrokinetic system: for caries removal and cavity preparation. *JAm Dent Assoc 2000;131(6):777-85.*

31. **Hegde VS, Khatavkar RA.** A new dimension to conservative dentistry: Air abrasion. *J Conserv Dent 2010;13(1):4-8.*

32. **Holmgren CJ, Roux D, Domejean S.** Atraumatic restorative treatment (ART) An a minima approach to the management of carious lesions. *Real Clin 2011;22(3):245-56.*

33. **Hormiere J.** Instruments d'optique ophtalmique. *Paris: Lavoisier, 2010.*

34. **Huth KC, Paschos E, Brand K, Hickel R.** Effect of ozone on non-cavitated fissure carious lesions in permanent molars. A controlled prospective clinical study. *Am JDent 2005;18(4):223-8.*

35. **Ie YV, Verdonschot EH, Schaeken MJ, Van't Hof MA.** Electrical conductance of fissure enamel in recently erupted molar teeth as related to caries status. *Caries Res 1995;29(2):94-9.*

36. **Jablonski-Momeni A, Klein SM.** In-vivo performance of the CarieScan pro device for detection of occlusal dentine lesions. *Open Accs J Sci Tech 2015;3:1-6.*

37. **Jain K, Bardia A, Geetha S, Goel A.** Papacarie: A Chemomechanical Caries Removal Agent. *IJSS Case Rep Rev. 2015;1(9):57-60.*

38. **Javier-Moder RM, Kuntz JL.** Occupational bone diseases. *Rev Rhum 2003;70(12):1062-9.*

39. **Jayarajan J, Janardhanam P, Jayakumar P.** Efficacy of CPP-ACP and CPP-ACPF on enamel remineralization-An in vitro study using scanning electron microscope and DIAGNOdent®. *Indian JDentRes 2011;22(1):77-82.*

40. **Jia L, Stawarczyk B, Schmidlin PR, Attin T, Wiegand A.** Effect of caries infiltrant application on shear bond strength of different adhesive systems to sound and demineralized enamel. *JAdhes Dent 2012;14(6):569-74.*

41. **Katakam D,Priyadarshini S, Raghu R, Shetty A, Premlatadevi T, Cherukuri S.** An in vitro comparative evaluation of enamel microhardness in soft drinks, CPP-ACP, amine fluoride and sodium fluoride with functionalized tricalcium phosphate. *JEvolutionMedDent Sci 2017;6(4):273-7.*

42. **Kornblit R, Trapani D, Bossù M, Muller-Bolla M, Rocca JP, Polimeni A.** The use of Erbium: YAG laser for caries removal in paediatric patients following minimally invasive dentistry concepts. *Eur J Paediatr Dent 2008;9(2):81-7.*

43. **Kronenberg O, Lussi A, Ruf S.** Preventive effect of ozone on the development of white spot lesions during multibracket appliance therapy. *Angle Orthod2009; 79(1):64-9.*

44. **Lam A, Tramba P.** Sono-dentistry, what else? *InfDent. 2011;34:32-5.*

45. **Lasfargues JJ, Louis JJ, Kaleka R.** Classifications of carious lesions from Black to the current concept by sites and stages. *EMC-Odontologie 2006:1-19 [Article 23-069-A-10].*

46. **Lasfargues JJ, Colon P, Lambrechts P.** Conservative and restorative dentistry: A global medical approach. *Paris :CdP, 2009.*

47. **Lussi A, Hellwig E, Klimek J.** Fluorides - Modes of action and recommendations for use. *Schweiz Monatsschr Zahnmed 2012;122:1030-6.*

48. **LussiA, Schaffner M.** Diagnosis and treatment of caries. *Forum MedSuisse 2002;8:166-70.*

49. **Lussi A, Schaffner M.** Evolutions in restorative odontology. *Paris: Quintessence International, 2013.*

50. **Mackenzie L, Banerjee A.** Minimally invasive direct restorations: a practical guide. *Br Dent J2017;223(3):163-71.*

51. **Magnien-Grenier B.** Should you go for air abrasion? *Independent. 2003;1:40-7.*

52. **Mallet JP, Foxcroft R.** Microdentistry and optical systems. *Rev Odontostomatol 2002;31:83-107.*

53. **Manoharan V, Sivanraj AK.** Dental ozone - A revolution in pediatric dentistry. *Int JSci Res 2018;7(2):69-71.*

54. **Manton DJ.** Diagnosis of the early carious lesion. *Aust Dent J2013;58:35-9.*

55. **Marinho VC.** Evidence-based effectiveness of topical fluorides. *Adv Dent Res 2008;20(1):3-7.*

56. **Maru VP, Shakuntala BS, Nagarathna C.** Caries removal by chemomechanical (Carisolv™) vs rotary drill: A systematic review. *Open Dent J 2015;9:462-72.*

57. **Matalon S, Feuerstein O, Calderon S, Mittleman A, Kaffe I.** Detection of cavitated carious lesions in approximal tooth surfaces by ultrasonic caries detector. *Oral Surg Oral Med Oral Pathol Oral Radiol Endod 2007;103(1):109-13.*

58. **Mentouri A, Bakli N, Belgharbi I, Rachid SID.** Caries eviction by a non-invasive method: The Carisolv® system. *Fac Med 2016;4(1):31-5.*

59. **Meyer-LueckelH, Paris S.** Progression of artificial enamel caries lesions after infiltration with experimental light curing resins. *Caries Res 2008;42(2):117- 24.*

60. **Millar BJ, Hodson N.** Assessment of the safety of two ozone delivery devices. *JDent 2007;35(3):195-200.*

61. **Miller C, TenCate JM, Lasfargues JJ.** Remineralization of carious lesions (1).The essential role of fluorides. *Real Clin 2004;15:249-61.*

62. **Mital P, Mehta N, Saini A, Raisingani D, Sharma M.** Recent advances in detection and diagnosis of dental caries. *JEvo MedDent Sci 2014;3(1):177-91.*

63. **Mueller J, Yang F, Neumann K, Kielbassa AM.** Surface three-dimensional topography analysis of materials and finishing procedures after resinous infiltration of subsurface bovine enamel lesions. *Quintessence Int 2011;42(2):135-47.*

64. **Murakami C, Bonecker M, Corrêa MSNP, Mendes FM, Rodrigues CRMD.** Effect of fluoride varnish and gel on dental erosion in primary and permanent teeth. *Arch Oral Biol 2009; 54(11):997-1001.*

65. **Néri JD, Lomba E, Karam AM, de Almeida Reis SR, Marchionni AM, Medrado AR.** Ozone therapy influence in the tissue repair process: A literature review. *J Oral Diagn 2017;2(1):1-6.*

66. **Neumeyer S, Gernet W.** Wissenschaft-Minimal-Invasive Praparationstechnik. *ZWR-Das Deutsche Zahnarzteblatt 2001;110(3):130-3.*

67. **Nhu NV, Hong TP, Le AQ, Minh ST, Thu PN.** The effect of casein phosphopeptide-amorphous calcium fluoride phosphate on the remineralization of artificial caries lesions: an in vitro study. *JDent Indones 2017;24(2):45-9.*

68. **Ntovas P, Doukoudakis S, Tzoutzas J, Lagouvardos P.** Evidence provided for the use of oscillating instruments in restorative dentistry: A systematic review. *Eur JDent 2017;11(2):268-73.*

69. **Paris S, Meyer-Lueckel H.** Masking of labial enamel white spot lesions by resin infiltration--A clinical report. *Quintessence Int. 2009; 40(9):713-8.*

70. **Peruchi C, Santos-Pinto L, Santos-Pinto A, Barbosa e Silva E.** Evaluation of cutting patterns produced in primary teeth by an air-abrasion system. *Quintessence Int 2002;33(4):279-83.*

71. **Pitts NB, Ekstrand KR.** International caries detection and assessment system (ICDAS) and its international caries classification and management system (ICCMS)-methods for staging of the caries process

and enabling dentists to manage caries. *Community Dent Oral Epidemiol 2013;41(1):41-52.*

72. **Pretty IA.** Caries detection and diagnosis: Novel technologies. *JDent 2006;34(10):727-39.*

73. **Reynolds EC.** Casein phosphopeptide-amorphous calcium phosphate: the scientific evidence. *Adv Dent Res 2009;21(1):25-9.*

74. **Santos-Pinto L, Peruchi C, Marker VA, Cordeiro R.** Effect of handpiece tip design on the cutting efficiency of an air abrasion system. *Am J Dent 2001;14(6):397-401.*

75. **Schelle F, Polz S, Haloui H, Braun A, Dehn C, Frentzen M, Meister J.** Ultrashort pulsed laser (USPL) application in dentistry: basic investigations of ablation rates and thresholds on oral hard tissue and restorative materials. *Lasers MedSci 2014;29(6):1775-83*

76. **Schneider H, Albert M, Busch M, Haefer M, Jentsch H.** Infiltration of natural caries lesions with monomer under simulated conditions of the oral cavity. *JDent Res 2008;24(3):164.*

77. **Sghaier T, Ben Abdallah MA.** Comparative study of the physicochemical composition of twenty brands of packaged water marketed in Tunisia. *JNew Sci Agri Biotech 2018;56(3):3671-86*

78. **Singh S, Singh DJ, Jaidka S, Somani R.** Comparative clinical evaluation of chemomechanical caries removal agent Papacarie® with conventional method among rural population in India: in vivo study. *Braz J Oral Sci 2011;10(3):193-8.*

79. **Sorvari R, Meurman JH, Alakuijala P, Frank RM.** Effect of fluoride varnish and solution on enamel erosion in vitro. *Caries Res 1994;28(4):227-32.*

80. **Stroumza JM.** Contribution of lasers in dentistry. *Actual*

Odontstomatol 2015;272:2-14.

81. **Tao S, Li L, Yuan H et al.** Erbium laser technology vs traditional drilling for caries removal: a systematic review with meta-analysis. *J Evid Based Dent Pract 2017;17(4):324-34.*

82. **TasseryH, Slinami A, Acquaviva M, Cautain C, Beverini MN, Terrer E.** Diagnostic methodology in cariology. Contribution of new technologies. *Real Clin 2014;25(2):129-37.*

83. **Tassery H, Victor JL, Coudert G, Brouillet JL, Koubi S.** Dentisterie restauratrice a minima. *EMC - Odontologie 2006:1-13 [Article 23-145-A-05].*

84. **Thakre G, Reddy MG, Kulkarni M, Chaudhari S, Vidhale S.** Histobacteriological evaluation of advancing front of carious dentin: Excavation done with and without using caries disclosing dye. A comparative in vitro study. *JDent Res Sci Develop 2015;2(2):22-5.*

85. **Tiwari S, Avinash A, Katiyar S, Iyer AA, Jain S.** Dental applications of ozone therapy: A review of literature. *Saudi JDent Res 2017;8(1-2):105-11.*

86. **Wu J, Donly ZR, Donly KJ, Hackmyer S.** Demineralization depth using QLF and a novel image processing software. *Int JDent. 2010;2010:1-7.*

87. **Yanikoglu FÇ, Õztürk F, Hayran O, Analoui M, Stookey GK.** Detection of natural white spot caries lesions by an ultrasonic system. *Caries Res 2000;34(3):225-32.*

88. **Zero DT, Fontana M, Martinez-Mier EA et al.** The biology, prevention, diagnosis and treatment of dental caries: scientific advances in the United States. *J Am Dent Assoc 2009;140:25-34.*

89. **Zhegova GG, Rashkova MR, Yordanov BI.** Perception of Er-YAG laser dental caries treatment in adolescents-A clinical evaluation. *JIMAB Ann Proceed Sci Papers 2014;20(1):500-3.*

Internet references :

90. **Azogui-Levy S, Baillon-Javon E, Beley G.** Strategies for preventing dental caries [Online]. *[Accessed 10/07/2018], Available from URL: https://www.has-sante.fr/portail/upload/docs/application/pdf/2010-10/corriges_rapport_cariedentaire_version_postcollege-10sept2010.pdf*

91. **Castot A, Rouleau-Quenette A, Broca O, Rebiere I.** Use of fluordin the prevention of dental caries before the age of 18 [Online]. *[Accessed 10/07/2018], Available from URL: https://ansm.sante.fr/var/ansm_site/storage/original/application/7db1d82db 7f5636b56170f59e844dd3a.pdf*

92. **Dental Achat.** The specialist for your dental products and materials [Online]. *[Accessed 14/10/2018], available from URL: https://www.dentalachat.com/*

93. **GC.** GC Tooth Mousse, GC Mi Paste Plus and GC Dry Mouth [Online]. *[Accessed 05/08/2018], Available from URL: https://www.tooth- mousse.fr/ F_frame.html?https://www.tooth-mousse.fr//*

94. **Icon® DMG.** Infiltration of caries [Online]. *[Accessed 13/05/2018], Available from URL: http://docplayer.fr/20248369-Traiter-les-taches-blanches-stopper-les-caries-debutantes-icon-l-infiltration-des-caries.html*

95. **Martin JR.** G.V. Black's classification of caries [Online]. *[Accessed 11/03/2018], Available from URL: https://dentodontics.com/2015/02/26/g-v-blacks-classification-of-carious-lesions/*

96. **Rey G.** The principle of the Laser [Online]. *[Accessed 14/10/2018], Available from URL: https://journal-stomato-implanto.com/content/le-principe-du- laser-0*

97. **Rocha L, Garcez J, Torres O.** Micro-invasive treatment with resin infiltration technique [Online]. *[Accessed 04/11/2018], Available from URL: https://ipj. quintessenz. de/poster946.pdf*

98. **USAF Dental Evaluation, Consultation Service.** Airbrator Air Abrasion Handpiece [Online]. *[Accessed 22/08/2018], Available from URL:*

https://www.airforcemedicine.af.mil/Portals/1/Documents/DECS/Product_Ev al uations/Equip/Air_Abrasion/Airbrator_Air_A brasion.pdf

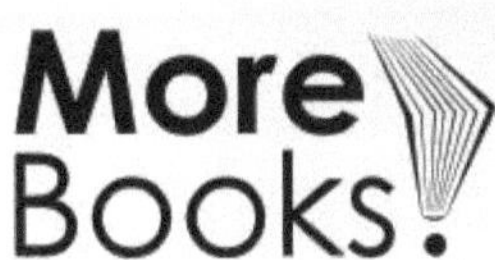
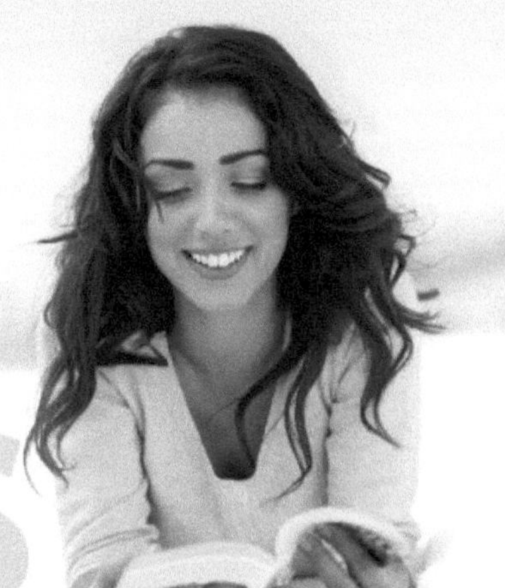

I want morebooks!

Buy your books fast and straightforward online - at one of world's fastest growing online book stores! Environmentally sound due to Print-on-Demand technologies.

Buy your books online at
www.morebooks.shop

Kaufen Sie Ihre Bücher schnell und unkompliziert online – auf einer der am schnellsten wachsenden Buchhandelsplattformen weltweit! Dank Print-On-Demand umwelt- und ressourcenschonend produzi ert.

Bücher schneller online kaufen
www.morebooks.shop

info@omniscriptum.com
www.omniscriptum.com

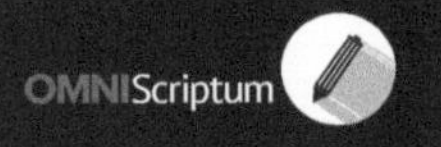

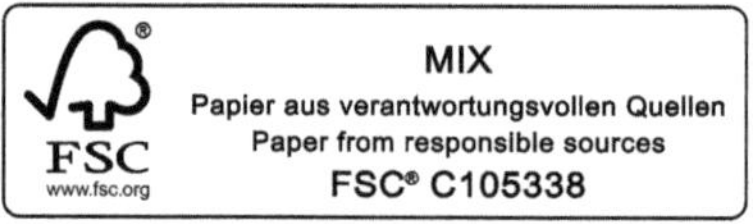

Printed by Books on Demand GmbH, Norderstedt / Germany